CW01035418

Hypnosis for Inner Conflict Resolution

Introducing Parts Therapy

C. Roy Hunter MS FAPHP

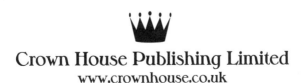

Crown House Publishing Limited
www.crownhouse.co.uk

First published by

Crown House Publishing Ltd
Crown Buildings, Bancyfelin, Carmarthen, Wales, SA33 5ND, UK
www.crownhouse.co.uk

and

Crown House Publishing Company LLC
6 Trowbridge Drive, Suite 5, Bethel, CT 06801, USA
www.crownhousepublishing.com

First published 2005, Reprinted 2006, 2008, 2010, 2012 and 2015.

British Library Cataloguing-in-Publication Data
A catalogue entry for this book is available from the British Library

ISBN: 978-1904424600

LCCN: 2004111439

Printed and bound in the USA

Contents

Acknowledgments v

Foreword by Terence Watts...vii

Introduction...ix

Chapter 1   Overview..1
       1.1 What is parts therapy? 2
       1.2 When is parts therapy appropriate? 4
       1.3 Who will most likely respond? 5
       1.4 Why is client-centred parts therapy effective? 5
       1.5 Variations of parts therapy 6
          1.5.1 Ego state therapy 6
          1.5.2 Voice dialogue 7
          1.5.3 Inner-child work 8
          1.5.4 Subpersonalities 9
          1.5.5 Other variations 9

Chapter 2   **Charles Tebbetts: Parts Therapy Pioneer** 13
       2.1 Who was Charles Tebbetts? 13
          2.1.1 Parts therapy pioneer 15
          2.1.2 Article written by Charles Tebbetts 16
       2.2 Important updates 19

Chapter 3   **Important Background Information** 23
       3.1 What is client-centred hypnosis? 24
       3.2 The four primary hypnotherapy objectives 24
          3.2.1 Objective 1: Suggestion and imagery 25
          3.2.2 Objective 2: Discovering the cause 26
          3.2.3 Objective 3: Release 27
          3.2.4 Objective 4: Subconscious relearning 28
          3.2.5 Additional comments 29
       3.3 Which hypnotherapy objectives can parts
          therapy fulfill? 30
       3.4 Why training in regression therapy is a
          prerequisite 30
          3.4.1 Inappropriate leading 32
       3.5 Psychodynamics and ideomotor responding 33
          3.5.1 Let the client choose the finger
          responses 35

3.5.2 Seven important questions
(psychodynamics) 36

Chapter 4   **Proper Preparation** **39**
4.1 Explain parts therapy to the client 39
4.2 Hypnotize and deepen appropriately 42
4.3 Establish a safe place 43
4.4 Establish (or confirm) finger responses 45
4.5 Verify hypnotic depth 45
4.6 Know the eleven-step process 48
4.7 Additional comments 49

Chapter 5   **The First Four Steps** **51**
5.1 The risk of imagery in parts therapy 51
5.2 Step 1: Identify the part 52
5.3 Step 2: Gain rapport 53
5.4 Step 3: Call out the part 55
5.5 Combining Steps 1–3 56
5.6 Sample scripts 58
5.6.1 Calling out the conflicting part 58
5.6.2 Calling out the motivating part 59
5.7 Step 4: Thank it for emerging 60
5.8 Reviewing Steps 1–4 61
5.9 Possible detours 61

Chapter 6   **The Important Fifth Step: Discover Its Purpose** **65**
6.1 Why should a part choose a name or title? 65
6.2 Ask the "W" questions 67
6.2.1 What ...? 68
6.2.2 How ...? 70
6.2.3 Why ...? 71
6.2.4 When ...? 73
6.2.5 Who ...? 74
6.2.6 Where ...? 74
6.2.7 John's sample session 74
6.3 Possible detours 75
6.4 Avoid inappropriate leading 76
6.5 Sample scripts 78
6.6 Important advice from Charles Tebbetts 80
6.7 Parts that use finger responses 82

Chapter 7   **Let the Mediation Begin** **85**
7.1 Step 6: Call out other parts as appropriate 85
7.1.1 Calling out the motivating part 85
7.1.2 Calling out the conflicting part 88
7.1.3 Calling out a third part 88
7.1.4 Calling out a part repeatedly 89

7.2 Step 7: Mediate and negotiate 89
   7.2.1 Listen and mediate 90
   7.2.2 How to negotiate 91
7.3 Possible detours 93
   7.3.1 The wrong part emerges 94
   7.3.2 Dealing with mistrust 94
   7.3.3 When parts refuse to negotiate 96
   7.3.4 Negative or uncooperative parts 98

Chapter 8   **Terms of Agreement** **101**
8.1 Step 8: Ask parts to come to terms of agreement 101
   8.1.1 What to ask 102
   8.1.2 Possible detours 104
   8.1.3 Calling out the inner wisdom 105
8.2 Step 9: Confirm and summarize terms of
      agreement 106
   8.2.1 Possible detours 108

Chapter 9   **The Final Steps** **111**
9.1 Step 10: Give direct suggestion as appropriate 111
9.2 Step 11: Integrate the parts 113
9.3 Give additional suggestions and/or guided
      imagery 116
9.4 Concluding the session 117

Chapter 10   **The Typical Session** **119**
10.1 John: Weight reduction 119
10.2 Outline of parts therapy session 125

Chapter 11   **Sample Sessions** **127**
11.1 The smoker 127
11.2 A smoky mirror 134
11.3 Unexpected cause 135
11.4 Career compromise 139
11.5 Getting big 141
11.6 Big protection 142
11.7 Professional confidence 143
11.8 This one is personal 144
11.9 Sweet tooth 145
11.10 The rose 145

Chapter 12   **Potential Pitfalls and Other Concerns** **147**
12.1 Advance explanation not given 147
12.2 Assuming command and giving orders 148
12.3 Calling out too many parts 150
12.4 Creating new parts 151
12.5 Criticizing a part 152

12.6 Freezing or immobilizing a part 152
12.7 Getting sidetracked 153
12.8 Multiple personality disorder 154
12.9 Alleged entities 156
  12.9.1 What if the part claims to be an entity? 156
  12.9.2 What if the client wants a part dismissed? ..159
  12.9.3 The therapist initiates the decision 160
12.10 Skipping steps 163
12.11 Taking sides with the dominant part 164
12.12 Other concerns 164

Chapter 13   **New Frontiers: The Undiscovered Country** **167**
13.1 Experts visit new frontiers 167
13.2 Seeking resolution from a spiritual part 168
  13.2.1 The Road 169
  13.2.2 Light for the life path 170
  13.2.3 Awareness of life path 170
  13.2.4 Divine guidance 171
13.3 Unresolved past grief 174
  13.3.1 Resolution with hypnotic regression 175
  13.3.2 Gestalt role-play in a sacred place 175
  13.3.3 The diamond 176
13.4 Healing the soul 177
13.5 Exploring spiritual potential—and more 180

Bibliography..**183**

Index **185**

Acknowledgments

This book is written for all therapists and hypnosis students who seek to empower their clients with client-centered hypnosis. It is dedicated to the memory of the late Charles Tebbetts, whose legacy to the hypnotherapy profession will, in my opinion, influence it for decades to come. Though his work with parts therapy evolved from the work of Paul Federn, I consider Charles Tebbetts to be one of the fathers of client-centered parts therapy. I appreciate that he trusted me to continue his work.

My deepest appreciation also goes into print for the professional acknowledgment received from Gil Boyne of the American Council of Hypnotist Examiners, and from Dwight Damon of the National Guild of Hypnotists. The professional awards they gave me in the name of Charles Tebbetts mean more to me than I can put into words.

Additionally, I wish to give special acknowledgment to certain fellow professionals and friends who have supported, promoted, or endorsed my work in recent years. Some have greatly influenced the completion of this parts therapy book either directly or indirectly, with a few providing input for the final manuscript. I mention them in alphabetical order (omitting titles and academic credentials): Cal Banyan, Randal Churchill, Don Gibbons, Kevin Hogan and Terence Watts.

Other people supportive of my work could be listed here, including professionals and friends who have sponsored my workshops, as well as hypnosis instructors teaching my course. Numerous students and professionals attending my presentations over the years have also encouraged me to write an entire book dedicated to parts therapy, and they have my gratitude for motivating me to make this book a reality. You know who you are, and I thank you.

I also express my heartfelt thanks to those who permitted me to include their session notes in the latter chapters of this book. My sincere hope is that many others may benefit from what you generously permitted me to share.

Last but not least, I appreciate Jo-Anne for her patience during the many evenings I worked late writing this book. While a part of me wanted to enjoy those evenings with her, another part motivated me to finish this book earlier than my publisher's expectations. The result is in your hands.

Foreword

To keep alive a specific work of a Master without destroying its credibility by seeking possession takes a man of extraordinary integrity and honour. It also needs a supremely effective vehicle to address the task in such a way as to inspire without sensationalising, promote without selling, and enlighten without seeming to patronise.

The Master is Charles Tebbets, the specific work is PARTS therapy, and the man is Roy Hunter, once a protégé of Tebbets and now a Master in his own right. The vehicle is this book that is about to inspire and enlighten you, the fortunate reader.

There are two reasons why I am certain of these things. One is that I have been well and truly on the receiving end of the work, the second is that I have twice in recent years had the privilege of organising and sponsoring enormously popular PARTS workshops for Mr Hunter in the UK. It was on one of those occasions that I was fortunate enough to be the volunteer with whom Mr Hunter himself exercised his considerable skills. To be in such a "hot seat" was the most profound of experiences, successfully addressing issues that had lain dormant since my earliest formative years.

PARTS is an elegant therapy. It can look so easy and effortless that you could be forgiven for thinking that it is simply a natural process—and indeed it is, for it *actually uses* the conflicts that are ever present in our psyche to resolve the apparently irresolvable, to quieten the incessant and resource-draining demands created by our opposing desires.

We should not, however, be misled. A natural process it may be but we need to be taught how to use it wisely and skilfully if we are not to make a mess of things. We need to know *when* to use it if we are to get the best of it. In short, we need a teacher of consummate skill, total professionalism and knowledge based on vast experience—

and Mr Hunter more than fits the bill. To watch him work is akin to watching a world-class conductor with a wonderful symphony orchestra, picking out the smallest of instruments, the most subtle of sounds at just the right moment to allow them to come together in perfect unison.

He is the conductor; the instruments of the orchestra are the parts of the psyche that he brings into beautiful and perfect harmony.

There are many who claim skill with PARTS work but who have acquired it via circuitous routes that have drained much of its character and power. Now, at last, here is your chance to learn directly from one who has himself become an undisputed Master of the Art.

Terence Watts

Introduction

How often do people experience inner conflicts that inhibit success-ful attainment of important goals? Parts therapy may provide the answer.

Counselors and hypnotherapists often use proven techniques to help their clients change undesired habits and/or to achieve desired personal and professional goals. Yet, in spite of the best efforts of both client and therapist, unresolved inner conflicts often inhibit clients from attaining their ideal empowerment. Often smokers, after rejecting both direct and indirect suggestions to quit, can finally attain inner resolution through parts therapy. Likewise, numerous clients attempting to control eating habits often gain important insight about themselves after experiencing hypnotic inner-conflict resolution. Other inner conflicts can also be resolved even after clients fail to respond to common hypnotic techniques.

Increasing numbers of therapists around the world are discovering the benefits of parts therapy and its variations to help clients get past personal barriers, and it continues to grow in popularity. Other therapists employing variations of parts therapy often use different names, such as *ego-state therapy, submodalities, subpersonalities, voice dialogue*. Regardless of the label, this author believes this complex technique to be the most beneficial hypnotic technique available for helping clients resolve inner conflicts.

The late Charles Tebbetts, a hypnotherapy instructor who taught thousands of students during his life, promoted and taught hyp-notic inner-conflict resolution as *parts therapy*. Originally borrowing it from Paul Federn, this twentieth-century hypnosis pioneer evolved parts therapy into a client-centered approach that can be learned by almost any experienced hypnotherapist competently trained in the basic concepts of facilitating subconscious release and relearning. Blazing new trails inside a relatively new hypnotherapy profession that American psychologists labeled "lay hypnotism",

Tebbetts was inducted into the International Hypnosis Hall of Fame for Lifetime Achievement. His work with parts therapy played a significant role in that honor.

Referred to by many hypnotists as a "master teacher", Charles Tebbetts wrote *Miracles on Demand,* a book about parts therapy and other hypnotic techniques, which went out of print after his death in 1992. Before he died, he asked me to continue his work; and one of the first tasks was to put my mentor's work back into the printed page. Although famous for his work with parts therapy, Charlie taught a number of other hypnotic techniques. After I had added my own professional updates, the total work became a two-volume text: *The Art of Hypnosis: Mastering Basic Techniques* (2000), 3rd edition (Kendall/Hunt Publishing), and *The Art of Hypnotherapy* (2000), 2nd edition (Kendall/Hunt Publishing). When I first wrote *The Art of Hypnotherapy,* I devoted one lengthy chapter to parts therapy. This effective hypnotic technique was sprinkled into several other chapters, with considerable additional information packed into the rest of the text. Other books are available describing parts therapy or its variations, but little is available originating in the hypnotherapy profession that is dedicated to parts therapy.

Over the years, I've enjoyed the privilege of teaching parts therapy workshops at various hypnosis conventions and hypnosis schools on both sides of the ocean. Students thirsty for knowledge frequently ask me where they can find additional information, because they need more than what my older text provides regarding this complex technique. Most of the additional information available regarding parts therapy and its variations is written for psychotherapists and other healthcare professionals who might use hypnotherapy as an adjunct to their practice, with minimal information available for those who specialize in the use of hypnosis as their primary profession. This book is intended to help fill that gap.

My primary purpose in devoting an entire book to parts therapy is to provide a learning tool for both the teacher and student alike. I intend this to be a "how to" guidebook, containing step-by-step instructions for facilitating competent, client-centered parts therapy from start to finish. I'll share techniques to help the properly trained hypnotist know when to consider parts therapy for a client, as well as how to obtain good results.

While other therapists may take their clients down different paths, my own professional experience validates the benefit of following the steps described in this book. If you are a therapist using ego states therapy, voice dialogue, or any other variation of parts therapy, then consider what I present only if it adds to your proven program. I will not debate with successful results. However, if you are not already trained in a successful variation of parts therapy, my strong recommendation is that you closely follow the discipline presented in the chapters that follow.

This book guides you through effective steps in sequence, with scripts (where appropriate), and also reveals potential pitfalls in order to minimize the risk of falling into one. Occasionally, we may run into detours along the way, and I'll share ideas that have helped me get past the detours over the years. Additionally, the discipline I present here assumes that parts therapy is combined with hypnosis in order to maximize the probability of longer-lasting beneficial results. Rather than simply employing parts therapy with little or no hypnotic depth, my students facilitate *hypnotic inner-conflict resolution*. This requires deeper states of hypnosis, which increases the probability of long-term success.

Hypnosis instructors need this book if they plan to teach parts therapy, even if they only recommend this book to their students as reference. Additionally, because I update my own work, the reader who owns a copy of either of the first two editions of *The Art of Hypnotherapy* will discover some additional changes to my older instructions. I consider one of these changes to be very important, and explain why in Chapter 2.

In conformance with my established writing style, I frequently use first-person format. Also, I use simple language for easy reading. While the discipline for effective parts therapy is complex, I believe that easy reading makes the learning process easier. Client examples included will be changed sufficiently in details in order to protect client confidentiality, except where permission was given. My professional opinions stated in these chapters resulted from insight provided by both my own experience and that of others.

This book is dedicated to all competent professionals who wish to master client-centered parts therapy in order to help clients resolve inner conflicts.

Chapter 1
Overview

Parts therapy is based on the concept that our personality is composed of a number of various parts. Our personality parts are aspects of the subconscious, each with its respective jobs or functions of the inner mind. In other words, we tend to wear many different hats as we walk along the path of life.

Often we can be consciously aware of the various hats we wear as our personality parts influence our conscious actions. At work we get into the work mode, wearing the figurative hat of a dedicated worker; but the inner child, quiet while we are working, can't wait to come out and play at home. The professional whose demeanor is *strictly business* in the workplace may become an easygoing person with a silly sense of humor outside the workplace. The freshman attending a college class takes on the role of the student while listening attentively to the professor's lecture, but that same person could become loud and boisterous at a Saturday-night party.

Some people are accused of being "two-faced" because of displaying very obvious personality changes in different circumstances; but a change of face is not limited to a few. It is actually common to all of us to greater or lesser degrees. These personality changes may become more obvious during times of inner conflict, such as when a smoker trying to quit is caught in the act of lighting up.

Inner conflicts occur when we have two different parts of the subconscious pulling us in opposite directions. The smoker mentioned above might have a strong emotional desire to quit in order to have more money to spend on recreational activities, but another part of the mind provides pleasure in lighting up after meals or at other times. Every year countless numbers of smokers make New Year resolutions to quit, only to find their resolutions literally going up in smoke. This is only one example of many types of inner conflict. The most common one weighs heavily in the minds of millions: *weight loss.*

Over the years I've often said that diets work on the body, but not on the mind. Dieters keep on losing pound after pound, only to find the pounds they lose just pile back on. The never-ending quest for maintaining an ideal weight is one goal among many that drive millions of people to seek ways to overcome undesired habits. Increasing numbers of men and women around the world are now achieving weight management and other goals through a modality that in only a few short years has emerged from skepticism into public acceptance: *hypnosis*.

Does hypnosis help all the people all the time? While the obvious answer is no, even a partially trained hypnotist can help some of the people some of the time. A competently trained hypnotherapist can help many more clients successfully quit smoking and/or achieve other goals through common hypnotic techniques; but it is a fact that some of the people seeking help will have inner conflicts that are strong enough to prevent positive suggestions from providing any permanent benefit. These clients need more than hypnosis alone: they need parts therapy.

1.1 What is parts therapy?

Parts therapy is the process of calling out and communicating directly with any and all parts of the subconscious involved in helping a client achieve a desired result. The use of parts therapy for inner-conflict resolution normally involves mediation between the two primary parts in conflict, which I call the *conflicting part* and the *motivating part*. Many of my sessions involve calling out only two parts, but other parts do exist—and, occasionally, I call out more than two parts during a session.

The hypnotic state makes it easier to communicate with each part, and reduces the risk of interference from the analytical conscious mind. I employ and teach a process based on a discipline taught by the late Charles Tebbetts, and updated through my years of professional experience.

In previous writings, I started my discussion of parts therapy quoting the actual words of Charles Tebbetts, taken from *Miracles on Demand* (page 31; now out of print):

> In 1952, [Paul] Federn described Freud's ego state (id, ego and superego) as resembling separate personalities much like the multiple personalities illustrated in the celebrated case of "The Three Faces of Eve," but differing in that no one of them exists without the awareness of the others. I find, however, that in many cases different parts take complete control while the total individual is in a trance state of which she is unaware. A bulimic will experience time distortion while bingeing, eating for over an hour and believing that only five minutes have elapsed … Both personalities know that the other exists, but the first is unaware of the other's existence during the period of the deviant behavior.

My mentor believed that we all have various aspects of our personalities, which he sometimes called personality parts, but more often called ego parts. Some of the other names for ego parts are: *ego states, subpersonalities, selves,* and *developmental stages.*

His words continue:

> Surely, at some time you have thought, "Sometimes I feel that I want to do something. But at other times I think I would like to do the opposite." The well-adjusted person is one in whom the personality parts are well integrated. The maladjusted person is one in whom they are fragmented, and internal conflict exists.

My former instructor openly admitted that he borrowed aspects of parts therapy from other therapists and researchers, and then evolved his hypnotic application into a technique that effectively helps clients resolve inner conflicts. By teaching this complex technique in classes and workshops, Charles Tebbetts, I believe, made one of the most profoundly beneficial contributions to hypnotherapy in the twentieth century.

In a way, we could compare parts therapy to Gestalt, except that the client is role-playing different parts of his/her personality rather than role-playing other people. Competent use of parts therapy helps to discover the causes of problems, to release them, and then to facilitate subconscious relearning with the previously conflicting parts now integrated into a state of inner harmony.

The properly trained parts therapist is also a skilled hypnotist, employing parts therapy with a deeply hypnotized client, and then objectively talking to all the parts involved in attaining resolution of the client's concern. Often the best way to accomplish this is to find compromise, acceptance and resolution through negotiations and mediation. The entire process will be explored in depth later in this book.

1.2 When is parts therapy appropriate?

How often have you wanted to accomplish a goal or overcome an undesired habit, only to find your subconscious resisting? One part of your personality wants something, while another part of you doesn't want to pay the price.

A client experiencing such an inner conflict is an ideal candidate for parts therapy. The obvious clue would be evident in a client who says, "A *part* of me wants to get rid of this weight while *another* part wants to keep on eating!" The ego part desiring to be attractive is in conflict with the inner child (or some other ego part) wanting to enjoy eating, say, sweets. (There may be other reasons for the conflicting part to persist in overeating.) Parts therapy usually will uncover the cause(s), so that the therapist may facilitate inner-conflict resolution through a process similar to mediation.

Often the need for parts therapy may not be readily apparent. Therapists who practice diversified client-centered hypnosis learn how to fit the technique to the client rather than vice versa, and do not automatically use parts therapy with everyone. Most of my sessions begin with some positive suggestions designed to the client's specific benefits for achieving a desired goal, because an enjoyable first impression is lasting, and more likely to result in the client's keeping his/her next appointment. I also devote a session to teaching self-hypnosis as a way of reducing stress.

By the third or fourth session, if the client is resisting the positive suggestions, I'll choose an advanced hypnotic technique that seems appropriate for that particular client. Naturally, when an inner conflict is apparent, I choose parts therapy. When the appropriate technique is not so obvious, finger-response questions (explored in Chapter 3) usually help me to determine how to proceed.

While my primary motive for facilitating parts therapy is to help clients resolve inner conflicts, some trainers and authors use additional applications of parts therapy or its variations even in the absence of apparent inner conflicts.

1.3 Who will most likely respond?

The deeply hypnotized client is more likely to respond to parts therapy, while someone experiencing little or no hypnosis may easily resist the entire process, whether or not such resistance is apparent to the facilitator. Some therapists who use variations of parts therapy work with a client who is quite conscious. While many of their clients might respond with favorable results, a more analytical person might experience interference or resistance to the process, with some or most benefits being only temporary.

Also, the best way to empower the client to enjoy a more permanent resolution is to practice what I call *client-centered* parts therapy. This means that the answers and solutions to the client's concerns emerge from the client's own mind rather than from the mind of the therapist, including the name and purpose of each part that emerges.

1.4 Why is client-centered parts therapy effective?

In my professional opinion, it empowers the client when the resolution for the problem comes from that client instead of the therapist. Rather than give away his or her power to someone else who implants "spells" in the form of suggestions, the client discovers the best resolution by answering questions asked by the facilitator at appropriate times. (Later chapters in this book reveal what questions to ask, and when to ask them.)

Several years ago, a psychologist asked me to use parts therapy to help her resolve an inner conflict. Upon emerging from hypnosis, her first words were, "That solution was so simple, I wish I'd thought of it myself!" I quickly reminded her that the resolution had indeed come from her own mind, and not mine. She smiled and agreed, and acknowledged the value of parts therapy.

Client-centered parts therapy helps clients attain greater empowerment, because the power to change truly lies *within the client* rather than in the therapist. The facilitator of client-centered parts therapy has the task of identifying and calling out the right parts, asking the right questions, listening objectively, and following the discipline presented in this book.

1.5 Variations of parts therapy

Therapists have employed variations of parts therapy for decades. I'll briefly discuss several of them in this chapter section, starting with my favorite variation: *ego-state therapy*.

1.5.1 Ego state therapy

Pioneered by Dr John Watkins and Helen Watkins over a number of years, ego-state therapy has spread throughout the therapeutic world. John and Helen Watkins started writing about ego states in publications and books during the 1970s, adding an outstanding book in 1997 entitled, *Ego States: Theory and Therapy* (Watkins and Watkins, 1997). Gordon Emmerson PhD, takes ego-state therapy into the twenty-first century at warp speed with his important book, *Ego State Therapy* (2003), which is now required reading for my hypnotherapy students.

Emmerson believes that we use five to fifteen ego states throughout a normal week, and we have more available when needed. He goes beyond the use of ego states therapy for resolving inner conflicts, providing other therapeutic benefits as well. In my professional opinion, Emmerson's book is a "must read" for anyone practicing parts therapy. Besides calling out the ego states for inner-conflict resolution, Emmerson helps clients create a map of their own ego states. I find this process absolutely fascinating.

I believe that clients of any therapist who masters ego-state therapy as practiced and presented by Watkins or Emmerson should enjoy a high success rate. Emmerson believes that hypnosis makes ego-state therapy more powerful, which validates the teachings of Charles Tebbetts.

1.5.2 Voice dialogue

Anyone seriously searching for new ways of working with the inner mind will discover books about *voice dialogue*, another variation of parts therapy. Hal Stone PhD, and Sidra Stone PhD, explain voice dialogue in their voice-dialogue manual (1989), *Embracing Our Selves*. The client, in a manner that could compare to Gestalt therapy, plays the role of each part by changing chairs or positions (although changing chairs is optional). The therapist facilitates the dialogue and proceeds accordingly.

The Stones label the ego parts as *selves* or *subpersonalities*, and provide labels for the various other subpersonalities such as the protector/controller, the pleaser, and the perfectionist. Additionally, they provide some interesting discussion regarding when subpersonalities are created, including the possible origins of disowned selves, which they also call demonic energies.

A more contemporary book on voice dialogue is *The Voice Dialogue Facilitator's Handbook* by Miriam Dyak (1999). This later book presents Dyak's particular method of facilitating voice dialogue, with a step-by-step guide for those who wish to practice her approach. She has worked closely with Hal and Sidra Stone, and offers training programs.

Although voice dialogue is effective for many, my primary concern about it is the absence of a formal induction into hypnosis. With little or no trance state, the conscious mind is more easily able to allow analytical resistance. I know this from personal experience (as a client). The facilitator thought that he successfully helped me attain resolution to a concern as I moved from chair to chair; but I found my own conscious mind interfering greatly in the process. The benefits were temporary, and I believe the absence of hypnosis was the primary reason for my analytical resistance. Several of my students have reported similar experiences with voice dialogue over the years.

1.5.3 Inner-child work

John Bradshaw praised the work of Hal and Sidra Stone; but he considers the *selves* (or ego parts) to be developmental stages that remain intact, as discussed on page 217 of his book, *The Family: A Revolutionary Way of Self-Discovery*:

> Hypnotic age regression work clearly suggests that each of these developmental stages remains intact. There are an infant, a toddler, a pre-school and a school-age child in each of us, who feel and experience just as we did when we were children. There is an adolescent in us who feels and thinks just like we did in adolescence.

Bradshaw facilitates a group exercise in which he has a person close his/her eyes while others in the room give positive affirmations, with gentle music playing in the background. Does this sound like hypnosis? It *is*! He encourages his clients to meditate with inner imagery, and to love the inner child. He then takes his clients through all the "developmental stages" to find out whether the needs were met in each stage. Suggestions for positive change are given to each stage (or part of the inner child)—and he gets results. You decide whether or not this is a variation of parts therapy.

Others over the years have taught and written about how to work with the inner child. Whether or not parts therapy (or a variation) is even discussed, the simple act of working with an inner child must be based on the premise that we all have at least two parts: an inner adult and an inner child.

1.5.4 Subpersonalities

The concept of subpersonalities is presented in the very first paragraph of John Rowan's book (1993), *Discover Your Subpersonalities*:

> Are we just one person, just one self? Or do we have several little people inside us, all wanting different things? Why should we take it for granted that we have just one personality? Would it not make more sense to say that we are many? Maybe we have more than one centre within ourselves.

He goes on to suppose that our minds may be naturally divided into portions and phases, with earlier and later historical levels. Various zones and developmental strata might lead to many internal figures. Like most authors of similar books, he labels the various subpersonalities (or parts). Although somewhat analytical, his book is written for the novice. It is easy to read, with much useful information. It contains numerous exercises, along with some questionnaires for self-awareness.

I especially like Rowan's history of the variations of parts therapy covered in the 22nd and 23rd chapters of his book. That alone is sufficient for the serious student of parts therapy to invest in this book.

1.5.5 Other variations

Nancy J. Napier, a nationally known marriage and family therapist, also works with a variation of parts therapy. Her book (1990), *Recreating Your SELF: Help for Adult Children of Dysfunctional Families*, also gives examples of the origins of various personality parts. She calls them "protector" parts and "resource" parts, and provides some self-hypnosis scripts for identifying, cleansing and healing our various parts. She has researched through extensive written resources to back up her work, including Beahrs (1981) and Watkins and Watkins (1979).

A number of hypnotherapists use a variation of parts therapy called *conference room therapy*. Although it is similar to parts therapy in many ways, they use the imagery of a conference room. There are others who assume that subpersonalities are attaching entities that must be released rather than potentially productive parts that can be integrated or given new jobs.

Some variations involve *physical parts*. I have personally met and talked to a hypnotherapist who uses a variation of parts therapy by facilitating dialogue with various physical parts of the body. His clients role-play (as in Gestalt therapy) being the heart, the brain, the liver, the foot, the ear, etc. Apparently he gets results. David Quigley, founder of the Alchemical Hypnotherapy Institute, teaches a variation of parts therapy that is similar to that of Charles Tebbetts, but he seeks out specific parts that do specific jobs. Our two approaches are both different and compatible. Also, Kevin Hogan PhD, employs and teaches a variation of parts therapy that is similar to what I teach. He discusses this in his book, *The New Hypnotherapy Handbook* (2001).

I'm certain that other therapists practice additional variations of parts therapy somewhere around the world; but this book is intended to teach the step-by-step parts therapy process the way I practice it. Those who wish to explore all the variations may wish to start by reading the books referenced in this chapter (and for which publisher information is in the Bibliography) and do their own research. Besides using deep trance, another difference between my methods and that of most variations is that I do not label the parts. Instead, each emerging part gives me a name or title, which often provides important insight. Additionally, this is more client-centered than looking for a specific part (such as a *controller* part), which could cause parts to emerge that may be irrelevant to the therapy.

Although other variations of parts therapy may be effective for some people, I prefer to practice and teach this valuable hypnotherapeutic technique similar to the way Tebbetts taught it; but my experience has caused me to make some important updates to his teachings through the years. Certainly, Charles Tebbetts was not the first therapist to ever employ a variation of parts therapy; but in my opinion he evolved it to a client-centered approach. That makes him a pioneer.

Over my years of practice, I've modified his work to keep up with changing times. The next chapter discusses the most important updates, and provides a brief glimpse of Charles Tebbetts, a pioneer of parts therapy.

Chapter 2
Charles Tebbetts
Parts Therapy Pioneer

Hypnotherapists around the world know the name of Charles Tebbetts, but few know very much about his background. Although this chapter is not essential to understanding the effective use of parts therapy, I include it for the benefit of those interested in the life and work of this important pioneer of parts therapy. Additionally, I include this out of respect for my late mentor and personal friend, and out of respect for his widow, still living as these pages are written.

Much of the content of this chapter is based on what Tebbetts wrote in his book, *Miracles on Demand*, as well as information shared with me personally by my late mentor, who asked me to call him Charlie. Additionally, I will discuss a few important updates to his teachings as a result of my own professional experience with parts therapy.

2.1 Who was Charles Tebbetts?

Charles Tebbetts grew up in the Midwest. He lost his father when he was only fourteen. Although his mother wanted him to attend college and become a psychiatrist, Charlie's involvement with music interrupted the career she planned for him. Shortly after graduating from high school, he started playing for a jazz band. Young Tebbetts traveled throughout the eastern half of the United States, finally ending up playing for an orchestra at a vaudeville theater.

In 1927, this young saxophone player witnessed a stage hypnotist show five nights weekly for several months, and memorized the act. One night, the hypnotist drank excessively once too often, and was unable to perform. Meanwhile, the observant and curious musician, who studied the performer's techniques thoroughly, volunteered to provide the entertainment that night. The owner became so impressed that he replaced the alcoholic hypnotist with his saxophone player, and thus began the long hypnotic career of Charles Tebbetts.

Initially, the young Tebbetts devoted himself to the entertainment side of hypnosis. After many months, a doctor (who was a friend of the family) saw him perform one night in Beatrice, Nebraska, his mother's hometown. The physician persuaded the young hypnotist to work with him and with his patients. After considerable experiments, the doctor learned the art of hypnosis himself; but skepticism among his peers caused the physician to swear Charlie to silence, and they parted ways. Meanwhile, his mother was deeply disappointed, and urged her son to start another career. He chose advertising.

Charlie's new career helped enhance his belief in the power of self-hypnosis, which motivated him to work with a jeweler manufacturing Walt Disney character charms. After negotiating a lucrative contract with Walt Disney, he moved to Hollywood. After getting involved with music again, he met the woman who became Joyce Tebbetts. Although continuing his work with advertising, Charlie wrote numerous songs, recorded by several well-known country-and-western singers. (Some of his hit records would eventually be displayed on the wall of his hypnosis school in Edmonds, Washington, years later.)

His work with art, music, and advertising helped to pay his bills, but Tebbetts continually remained involved with hypnosis as a side business, conducting occasional sessions and doing research. He considered himself to be a lifelong student of hypnosis, always studying the work of others and always reading.

Charles and Joyce Tebbetts made their home in Southern California for a number of years. He eventually learned about Gil Boyne's work with hypnosis, and they met in 1970. Tebbetts liked the way Boyne taught and promoted hypnosis, and chose to attend Gil's school to learn more. They became personal friends, and soon Charlie started practicing out of Gil's facility. He later opened an office in Brentwood, and sold his advertising business.

After suffering a paralyzing stroke, Charlie first used self-hypnosis to regain his ability to talk, and then to walk once again. This experience inspired him to write *Self-Hypnosis and Other Mind Expanding Techniques*, which is available to this day.

Eventually, Charles and Joyce moved to Washington State to establish their own hypnosis training institute, as well as a state chapter of the American Council of Hypnotist Examiners. At his school in Edmonds, Charlie actively taught and promoted parts therapy to other professionals and to advanced students of hypnosis.

Although Charles Tebbetts always agreed with Gil Boyne over the need for competent training in hypnosis, he eventually broke away and formed his own organization, the Hypnotist Examining Council International (which eventually merged with the National Guild of Hypnotists). You may still obtain a copy of Charlie's self-hypnosis book either from Westwood Publishing or from Amazon.com.

During the late 1980s, Tebbetts reached the height of his fame throughout the entire hypnotherapy profession. Inducted into the International Hypnosis Hall of Fame for lifetime achievement, Charles Tebbetts is best remembered for his work with parts therapy.

2.1.1 Parts therapy pioneer

In the early 1980s, Tebbetts wrote the now out-of-print *Miracles on Demand*. Although this book contained a brief summary of his basic hypnosis training course, he devoted the majority of the book to scripts of actual therapy sessions facilitated in the classroom. Most of those sessions incorporated parts therapy. I personally witnessed a couple of the videotaped sessions that he included in his book.

When I attended his school in Edmonds in 1983, most of Charlie's demonstrations in the classroom involved the use of either regression therapy or parts therapy, and often both. Charlie liked parts therapy because of its ability to quickly help a client discover the core cause of a problem, which he called "hitting pay dirt". In his opinion, it was difficult to know what cause to release unless or until that cause was discovered (rather than diagnosed).

He openly admitted that he borrowed techniques from other professionals, and adapted them to his own hypnotic style. He taught that all hypnosis is self-hypnosis, and our job is to empower the client.

Tebbetts traveled to several hypnosis conventions to teach parts therapy to experienced therapists during his latter years. Then, while attending the annual convention of the National Guild of Hypnotists in August of 1992, he suffered a heart attack right at the convention site. He asked me to teach his parts therapy workshop on his behalf that day, and passed away in the middle of my presentation.

Called a "grandmaster teacher" by Dr John Hughes of the National Guild of Hypnotists, Charles Tebbetts taught thousands of students who came to him from all over the world. Out of the thousands he trained either at his school or in workshops over the years, I consider it an honor and a privilege that he asked me to continue his work. That being said, Charlie was a pioneer, and pioneers didn't always take the shortest route to their destinations, even though they arrived.

My own experience, combined with the experience of others, resulted in my updating the way that I teach and practice parts therapy. Before discussing them in this chapter, let's examine one of Charlie's last articles before his passing.

2.1.2 *Article written by Charles Tebbetts*

Charles Tebbetts entitled this article "The Use of Hypnotherapy in Integrating Disintegrated Personality Parts" (reprinted by Roy Hunter with prior written permission from the late author). The name of the individual mentioned in the letter was changed.

> In 1952 I read the works of [Paul] Federn and my experience to that date convinced me that he was on the right track.

He described Freud's ego states (id, ego, and super ego) as resembling separate personalities much like the multiple personalities in the celebrated case of "The Three Faces of Eve" but differing in that no one of them exists without the awareness of the others. I find, however, that in many cases different parts take control while the subject is in a light trance state of which he/she is unaware.

A bulimic will experience time distortion while bingeing when one of her parts takes over, and eat for over an hour believing only five minutes have elapsed. Another personality part then suffers shame and remorse. Both parts know that the other exists, but the first is unaware of the other's existence during the period of the deviant behavior.

Every individual is made up of parts, and the concept should always be explained to them before this type of therapy is used. Otherwise they might believe that they are multiple personalities. You might explain it to them in this matter:

Everyone is made up of various parts. Often a person might think, "I really want to take a vacation, but a part of me won't let me ..." or, "Part of me wants to get thin, but another part insists upon eating."

While the client is hypnotized, the therapist may ask to speak to the part that is causing the symptom, or he may call out the part that wants to get rid of it. Ask the part what name it wishes to be called. Ask the part that is causing the problem its reason for doing so. Ask the part that wishes to eliminate the symptom to talk to the offending part (by this time you know their names or titles) and plead its case.

Once the parts concept is accepted by the subconscious, other parts often speak up, and the therapist takes the role of *arbitrator*.

This is the point at which best results are assured by ignoring the permissive and indirect rules. I call this the "Great Debate." The therapist sides with the part that wants to eliminate the symptom and furnishes the logic the emotional parts have never considered. Rather than expecting a sick mind to cure itself, the therapist carries on a debate with the offending part or parts. The reason for the offending behavior or sickness is discussed and understood by all the parts, and now the therapist does the no-no and suggests a plan that the parts might agree to.

For example, I will cite the case of a one-session cure of migraine headaches and free floating anxiety. I called out the part that was causing the trouble, which called itself the power plant. It told me it was going to keep right on with its behavior, both to punish and protect Bob. I then asked the part that wanted to be free of the headaches to talk to the power plant and explain how it felt. Rather than addressing Joe, the power plant explained to me: "Bob is just like a little machine, thinking and planning, how to make more money. How to get ahead. He even plans and thinks in his sleep. I give him nightmares and awaken him with a headache so he can't work the next day, and I'm going to keep it up until he slows down."

I told Bob, "You heard what the power plant said. Maybe if you slow down he might quit punishing you."

Bob's answer was, "But I've tried to slow down. My main interest in life is planning moneymaking deals and investments. That is my hobby."

My answer was, 'Do you do much thinking and planning while you are having the headaches?"

Both parts continued to justify their actions until I said, 'The power plant is hurting your health. Maybe you could make a deal with him. Choose a certain number of hours a day for planning and thinking about getting ahead, and enjoy those hours to the fullest. Then relax and enjoy the rest of the time, the time you used to suffer with the headaches. You will get a lot more time to do your planning and you won't suffer with the headaches. Doesn't that plan sound better than nightmares, insomnia, and suffering?"

Bob agreed to follow my suggestions, and the power plant agreed to quit punishing him as long as he kept his agreement. Bob moved to the East Coast, and gave me a number of phone calls to tell me that one session had been a complete success. Following is the letter I received from him about a year after the session:

Dear Charles:

I would like at this time to sincerely thank you for your help in treating my headaches. It has been over a year now since your hypnosis treatment. After years of suffering, numerous medications, and doctor-recommended prescriptions which failed,

I am now virtually headache free with hypnosis. I practice
your self-hypnosis daily and find that I can not only control
headaches but improve other facets of my life.

Please accept my deepest thanks, and best wishes to you and
your charming wife Joyce.

Sincerely,

Bob

In closing, I will be glad to accept the honor of being a hypnotherapy heretic as long as I can document proof of continued success.

Charles Tebbetts

2.2 *Important updates*

Upon reading the above article closely, we notice that Charles
Tebbetts engaged in what he called the "Great Debate" (capitaliza-
tion his). He taught that the therapist should be an arbitrator who
sides in with the part wanting positive change. Note his own words
in the above article: "The therapist *sides with the part that wants to
eliminate the symptom* and furnishes the logic the emotional parts
have never considered" (emphasis mine).

I emphasize the importance of remaining objective, just as a
mediator would do while helping two people to resolve a conflict.

Let's examine the primary difference between arbitration and mediation. An arbitrator might listen objectively to both sides involved
in a conflict, but then he/she normally makes the decisions for each
party involved. By contrast, the *mediator* simply brings the conflicting sides together and facilitates open communication by encouraging each person involved to speak in turn and then to listen
appropriately. A skilled mediator can help the people involved in
conflict to come up with their own solutions by asking the right
questions.

While demonstrating parts therapy in his classroom, Tebbetts often acted like an arbitrator, but occasionally became more like a mediator. Although he obtained results both ways, Charlie was a debate champion in high school; thus he often engaged in debates with what he called the *offending* part (which I now refer to as the *conflicting* part). While I observed him facilitating session after session with results, I believe that he often obtained results where many of us might fail without his debating skills.

I personally like to avoid confrontation, and immediately took the more objective philosophy into my parts therapy sessions after completing his course, rarely engaging in any debates even when a part became obnoxious. My experience quickly validated the ability to get results without the risk of losing rapport with a part by arguing with it.

In 1990, one of my students chose to follow the teachings of Tebbetts to the letter, and paid a price after losing the "Great Debate" during a session. An offending part talked back to him, and the woman emerged immediately from hypnosis and failed to respond to any further attempts at induction. (More is written about this in Chapter 12.) I personally brought this fact to Charlie's attention, and he acknowledged that it would be the better path of wisdom for someone without debating skills to remain more neutral and objective.

To his credit, Tebbetts modified his position on debating with the offending part after this incident, and put more emphasis on remaining neutral and objective with all the parts. However, he did not live long enough to modify his teachings in his planned third edition of *Miracles on Demand* (which he never completed). He told me, "Hunter, my tapes show both my successes and my mistakes, but I still got results. Tell your students to do it your way if they don't have good debating skills."

To summarize, here are my three significant updates:

1. Be objective and neutral, and avoid debating with the parts.
2. Act as a mediator, not an arbitrator (updated since I wrote *The Art of Hypnotherapy*).
3. What Tebbetts called the "offending part" is now called the *conflicting part*.

Additionally, I organized the teachings of Charles Tebbetts into a step-by-step procedure presented in this book, from preparation to conclusion. I will take the reader through the entire parts therapy session from start to finish, including the appropriate procedures to use both before and after what I call the "eleven-step process". (Until 2003, I taught a twelve-step process, with suggestion and imagery representing the final step. However, just as a hypnotic induction precedes the parts therapy process, suggestion and imagery follow integration of the parts. This is explained in later chapters of this book.)

Some of my applications of the steps have also been updated through the years, which might become apparent to anyone who has either the first or second edition of my book, *The Art of Hypnotherapy*. One benefit of teaching parts therapy workshops to professionals is the combined wisdom of many decades of experience among the participants. Thus, I have occasionally updated my own teachings through the years. My philosophy is that we are all each other's teachers and students in the game of life, and the teacher who loses the ability to learn might also cease to be a good teacher.

Before exploring parts therapy, let's review some important background information presented in the next chapter.

Chapter 3
Important Background Information

The purpose of this chapter is to overview some important prerequisite information that will benefit both therapist and client alike. We need to understand some important concepts about hypnosis and hypnotherapy.

My opening statement in this chapter may not necessarily apply to those professional therapists who are experienced in the variations of parts therapy, but I believe that the information contained in this chapter becomes more important to those who incorporate hypnosis with parts therapy or its variations. My own students invest several months of training in the art of hypnosis before taking their first class on parts therapy for several reasons.

First, a hypnotherapist must master basic hypnotic techniques. An outstanding therapist could easily miss an opportunity to help someone make an empowering life change if the client is an analytical resister emerging from trance too soon. We should also know the difference between client-centered hypnosis and therapist-directed trance work.

Second, I provide a foundation for my students to build a multi-modality approach for their clients, incorporating the four primary hypnotherapy objectives. I'll discuss them in this chapter.

Third, one must understand how to competently facilitate regression therapy, because some clients spontaneously enter regression when we communicate with a part. The important difference between leading and guiding is too important to omit, although there is much more information about regression therapy than what appears in this chapter.

Additionally, there are a few other hypnotic techniques (such as ideomotor responding) that may often become quite useful in parts therapy, which will also be presented in this chapter. After defining client-centered hypnosis, I'll discuss *four hypnotherapy objectives*.

3.1 What is client-centered hypnosis?

Here is my explanation of the difference between client-centered hypnosis and therapist-directed trance work. During client centered hypnosis, the *client* comes up with the answers, provided the hypnotist skillfully uses the art of hypnosis to obtain those answers. This requires width and depth of training in the art of hypnosis.

Therapist-directed hypnosis is far more common around the world, and requires less hypnosis training, because the hypnotist determines whatever he/she thinks is the best solution for the client. Often the hypnotist simply uses a script book after just a few days of training, choosing a script to fit the client's concern. Generic scripts help some of the people some of the time, but often leave much undone.

3.2 The four primary hypnotherapy objectives

During the 1800s, our hypnotic pioneers primarily used *prestige suggestion* to obtain results. As the twentieth century approached, it became apparent that suggestion alone was insufficient to provide permanent benefit to many of the subjects hypnotized by our pioneers. Additionally, the scientific approaches fit the subject to the techniques rather than vice versa. One of the reasons Freud discarded hypnosis was that he grew tired of the monotonous sleep suggestions. Also, he did not believe that deep hypnotic states were necessary in order to achieve results. Perhaps if he had mastered the art of hypnosis, or learned to fit the technique to the client instead of fitting the client to the technique, we would have a totally different history of hypnosis and psychology—but let's deal with the current status of hypnosis today.

Certainly, hypnotic suggestion and imagery have proved their ability to help *some* of the people *some* of the time, but I believe that a competent hypnotherapist can help most of the people most of the time. We can accomplish this by building the therapeutic approach on a foundation of four primary hypnotherapy objectives:

- suggestion and imagery;
- discovering the cause;
- release; and
- subconscious relearning.

These four therapeutic objectives may be considered the cornerstones of effective hypnotherapy, especially where subconscious blocks are present, because *effective results often require fulfilling all four objectives*. In *The Art of Hypnotherapy*, I call these objectives "The Four Hypnotherapeutic Steps to Facilitate Change" (see Figure 1).

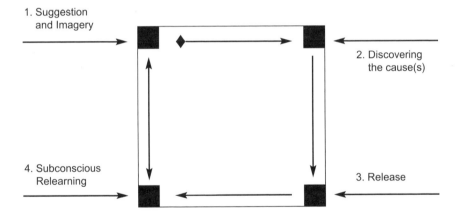

1. Suggestion and Imagery

2. Discovering the cause(s)

4. Subconscious Relearning

3. Release

Figure 1.

Now let's discuss each objective individually.

3.2.1 Objective 1: Suggestion and imagery

With a strong motivating desire, posthypnotic suggestions (direct or indirect) and imagery may be sufficient to provide lasting benefit to the client. Marketers of the hotel hypnosis seminars take advantage of this fact, and gather enough testimonials to attract thousands more to their traveling seminars. Without a strong desire, however, either the conscious or the subconscious may easily block the suggestions. How many people do you know who went to a hypnotist to stop smoking, only to start up again? (This is further evidence validating the belief that all hypnosis is self-hypnosis.)

When subconscious resistance exists (blocks), Objectives 2, 3, and 4 must all be used. The first objective then becomes the last one. This is why I consider these objectives to be the *four cornerstones* of successful hypnotherapy. They form the foundation for building a long-lasting success for your clients. Even when I know that all four objectives are necessary, I still start with the first one. By using suggestions to increase the motivating desire to change, the client is more likely to show up for any necessary subsequent sessions. Additionally, positive suggestion and imagery will usually leave a good impression of hypnosis, and first impressions are lasting.

3.2.2 Objective 2: Discovering the cause

If subconscious resistance exists, there is a reason. We may choose from among a variety of techniques that enable the subconscious to reveal the cause of a problem. Numerous books (in addition to mine) present various techniques for discovering the cause(s) of a client's problem. My favorites are ideomotor responding, hypnotic regression, and parts therapy.

Note that I do *not* attempt to determine the cause(s) myself: rather, I solicit the subconscious of my client to reveal the cause(s). If a therapist reaches a conclusion on the cause of a client's problem, and then employs hypnosis to validate that conclusion, there is a risk of subconscious confabulation. This would be *inappropriate leading*.

For example, if hypnotic regression is employed to "prove" that a client was abused, false memories may easily occur. Whether the therapist forms an opinion about the cause from analytical logic, professional conclusions, intuition, so-called psychic gifts, or religious beliefs (or a combination), what happens to the client if the therapist's opinion is incorrect? Preconceived opinions implanted by the therapist can taint the trance and take the client down the wrong path. (More will appear later on this topic.)

Even if the conclusion is a correct one, some other important cause might never emerge during the session. Unfortunately, such inappropriate leading happens in the offices of a number of therapists whose training in hypnosis is inadequate. The client-centered approach is to find a way to get the client's own mind to disclose the cause.

Once we discover the cause(s) of a client's concern, we must complete the next objective in order to reduce the risk that the client might buy back the problem.

3.2.3 Objective 3: Release

Awareness of the cause is not enough for everyone. Many clients will not be able to spontaneously release at a subconscious level unless asked to do so while experiencing deep hypnosis. During the hypnotic state, the relationship of the cause to the symptom is more easily established emotionally as well as intellectually. We may then use one or more hypnotherapy techniques to facilitate release. This often involves forgiveness of self and/or releasing others. Note that said release must be accomplished at a subconscious level, and not at the conscious level alone. While forgiving does not mean condoning, some clients may find the words "let it go" or "release it" to be more comfortable than "forgive". Regardless of the wording, it is usually very important that clients *forgive themselves*.

Several years ago, a woman saw me for a fear of flying. She experienced several hypnotic regressions with a psychologist, who would then bring her out of hypnosis and discuss the cause at a conscious level. He taught her to cope with her fear and live with it. I helped her to release it, so that she could comfortably get on a jet and fly anywhere in the world.

Speaking of fear of flying, some hypnotists take short cuts by trying to release a problem without discovering its cause. A salesman told me that he saw a hypnotist before flying to Australia, and she used a hypnotic releasing technique to have him release his fear without discovering the cause. He retained a degree of comfort on the outbound flight to Sydney, but experienced seventeen hours of severe anxiety on the return flight after his subconscious bought back the fear of flying.

Even if it is not disclosed to the therapist, the subconscious still must discover and identify the cause in order to release it. While I occasionally use a marvelous script written by the late Arthur Winkler that uses indirect suggestions to enable the subconscious to discover and release the cause of a problem, my client gives me a signal when this process is complete. In rare instances, the client's conscious mind might not be aware of the cause discovered by the subconscious; but finger responses can indicate when the inner mind discovers and releases the cause.

Do you think the first three objectives are enough? Think again. Numerous smokers have seen me over the years after quitting smoking previously with hypnosis, only to backslide weeks or months after their initial success. For that reason, we need to consider the next objective.

3.2.4 Objective 4: Subconscious relearning

If a smoker successfully quits through hypnosis, even after discovering and releasing the cause of the habit, his or her subconscious beliefs still influence the outcome. Clients who *believe* that they will start smoking again because of previous failures may indeed light up if they fantasize doing so often enough. In other words, to ensure success, the client must *believe* that the results will be lasting.

Numerous client-centered techniques can be used to facilitate adult understanding at a subconscious level, where it gets results. Once the subconscious mind *believes* that a problem is resolved, unencumbered by cause(s) previously discovered and released, the client is free to become self-empowered and achieve the desired goal. I ask the client to *imagine* fulfillment of his/her goal, and give additional suggestions that enable the client to *expect* long-term success.

After accomplishing the third objective, I often ask a client to verbalize his or her own relearning. Then I paraphrase their words back in the form of suggestions and imagery, which can be used to accomplish subconscious relearning. Notice the arrow going both directions between Objectives 1 and 4 on the diagram (Figure 1). Suggestions and imagery enhance subconscious relearning, and become much more powerful once the subconscious has discovered and released the cause(s) of a problem.

3.2.5 *Additional comments*

The numbers of various hypnotic techniques keep growing as new ones are invented and old ones are updated or modified. While it is not necessary to know every technique ever invented, the competent master of the art of hypnotherapy should have width and depth of training, as there is *no* technique that is effective enough to work for all the people all the time.

My students learn to evaluate the efficacy of any hypnotic technique on the basis of discerning which of the four hypnotherapy objectives it may accomplish. This provides a solid foundation for practicing diversified client-centered hypnosis and obtaining results without the necessity of asking my opinion on someone else's technique. If said technique works without risk to the client, *use* it; but learn to understand which objective(s) the technique accomplishes.

Over the years, clients have occasionally told me that another therapist failed to help them and then claimed the failure was because they were unable or unwilling to respond to hypnosis. Many hypnotists use only one modality (or program) that they attempt to use with all or most of their clients. Such hypnotists often get "certified" in a weekend training program that is too short to teach a multi-modality approach to hypnotherapy. This problem became prevalent throughout the 1980s and 1990s, as interest in hypnosis became widespread. Weekend certification programs still appeal to prospective students wanting to take short cuts to their training. Because the use of suggestion and imagery alone will help some of the people some of the time, graduates of the weekend certifications who have marketing skills often earn good money. Like the hotel hypnosis seminar marketers, they work with enough people to provide some credible testimonials from those who respond to suggestion and imagery alone.

While hypnotists using their pet programs do help some of the people some of the time, their success rates are often overstated. I wish that they would call themselves "hypnotists" rather than hypnotherapists, and refer resistant clients to competent hypnotherapists.

As I have stated many times in public and in print, the competent hypnotherapist can help most of the people most of the time by practicing diversified client-centered hypnosis. Expertise in parts therapy adds even greater width and depth to the toolbox of the competent hypnotherapist.

3.3 Which hypnotherapy objectives can parts therapy fulfill?

An entire hypnotic session that includes parts therapy will usually incorporate all four of the hypnotherapy objectives. However, the actual parts therapy process should always fulfill Objectives 2 and 3 (discover the cause, and release), and occasionally 4. The fourth objective (subconscious relearning) will be fulfilled after the final step of parts therapy if not before. Before awakening, suggestion and imagery (the first objective) will enhance subconscious relearning.

3.4 Why training in regression therapy is a prerequisite

My comments regarding hypnotic regression will be brief in this book (compared with what I could easily write), although they are important.

Spontaneous regressions often occur during parts therapy when the facilitator asks about a part's primary purpose as well as the origin of that purpose. In my professional opinion, nobody should even consider facilitating parts therapy without first receiving competent training in hypnotic regression therapy. There are important reasons for this opinion.

First, the facilitator must know how to guide a client through a hypnotic regression without implanting false memories. This requires the therapist to understand the important difference between leading and guiding. One must ask open-ended questions rather than closed ones, and avoid making assumptions. If you, the reader, are unclear on this issue, then I strongly suggest that you attend a workshop on regression therapy before you ever employ parts therapy, even if you already have a background in counseling. Also, note that we don't always remember things exactly as they happened, especially where emotions are involved. Ask two people who witness an emotional event to describe what happened, and you will often get two different versions of the same event. A client's perception of a past event may be a mixture of fact and fantasy. I inform my clients that we deal with subconscious perceptions rather than realities. In other words, the client may already have false memories blended with reality because of the emotions involved in a past event.

Second, the facilitator must know how to handle abreactions in a client-centered manner. If you don't know what an abreaction is, then you are not yet ready to facilitate a hypnotic regression. Some therapists are actually afraid of emotional discharges, and will bring a client out of hypnosis. Others encourage very strong emotions, with vulgar language or fantasies of violence to a perpetrator. Note that my position is that we should neither force nor inhibit abreactions during therapy. Instead, we should allow the client to express his or her emotions in whatever way is appropriate to that client. For some, it may be colorful language and/or sobbing loudly. For others, it may be one lone tear, or a sniffle, or just a few words spoken with feeling. If there is an absence of emotion, I invite the abreaction by asking, "How does that make you *feel*?" Then I listen to the response before proceeding. If the abreaction is intense, I'll either give suggestions to lessen the intensity, or guide the client through the abreaction quickly.

Third, the facilitator must know how to help the client release and/or reframe the original core cause of the afflicted part. Sometimes this may involve Gestalt role-play with the real or imagined perpetrator whose actions caused the problem in the first place. Also, I ask them to be ready to forgive themselves, and to release others who might have been involved. This release is also important as a preventive measure to reduce the risk that the client will accuse a relative of some alleged abuse that may have been misperceived.

After completing the regression, we must return the client to the parts therapy process before awakening him or her.

3.4.1 Inappropriate leading

Whenever a hypnotist helps a client attain a deep level of hypnosis, that client is in *rapport* with the hypnotist. If the level of trance is deep enough, that person may have an emotional desire to please the hypnotist, and provide whatever answers are expected. In other words, if uninformed hypnotists or psychotherapists use hypnotic regression to look for past abuse, they may often find it where it never existed—even if only in the imagination of both client and therapist alike.

Although I devoted one lengthy chapter of *The Art of Hypnotherapy* to regression therapy, there are other books available that cover far more information than I presented in my text. Unfortunately, most books on hypnotic regression emphasize past-life regressions; but two books worth reading are Randall Churchill's *Regression Hypnotherapy: Transcripts of Transformation* (2002) and Gil Boyne's *Transforming Therapy: a New Approach to Hypnotherapy* (1989). Another book, Alan Scheflin and Jerrold Lee Shapiro's *Trance on Trial* (1989), shows how inappropriate leading can occur during a hypnotic regression. Although the third book discusses the forensic aspects of hypnosis, the warning applies to any hypnotist or counselor employing hypnotic regressions: *avoid inappropriate leading*. If you project your own preconceived opinion into a client experiencing hypnotic regression, you will taint the trance—and who knows the possible consequences?

Before concluding this chapter section, I must quote the words of Emmerson from page 199 of his excellent book, *Ego State Therapy*: "There is no way to distinguish a false memory from a real one. Hypnosis cannot distinguish these memories and Ego State Therapy cannot distinguish them" (page 199).

My own personal experience as a client validates Emmerson's opinion. Some years ago an enthusiastic investigator of UFO incidents regressed me to a childhood out-of-body experience that happened after a scorpion bite had caused intense swelling and pain. When guiding me back to seeing the brilliant globe of light, she said, "Go through the light and tell me if you come out in a spaceship." As a hypnosis instructor, I knew afterwards that she was guilty of inappropriate leading, but the fantasy of being on a spaceship seemed real. Two years later I asked a competently trained hypnotist to regress me to the same incident. My subconscious then perceived the ball of brilliant light as an angel sent by God to heal my foot. The two conflicting memories of the same event seem equally as real and equally as fantasized.

Fortunately, it is not necessary for me to know which set of memories is correct. Perhaps the truth might be a combination of the two; or perhaps the globe of light might have been a hallucination caused by the scorpion's poison that was still in my body that night. Your guess is as good as mine is; however, this event helps me teach other therapists the importance of avoiding inappropriate leading.

Several minutes of proper hypnotic communication are more valuable than several months of resolution, for all parties concerned. If you have any concerns regarding your ability to facilitate a hypnotic regression, then my very strong recommendation is that you seek competent training in regression therapy before venturing into parts therapy or any of its variations.

3.5 Psychodynamics and ideomotor responding

This book would not be complete without devoting a few pages to ideomotor responding, also called finger-response questions. There are two primary reasons for including this information. First, the use of finger-response questions will often help to determine whether or not to use parts therapy with a client. Second (and rarely), a shy part sometimes uses finger responses for communication. I address the second reason later; but let's examine the first reason here.

Clients often fail to respond to positive suggestions, but don't make it obvious why. There may be one or more basic reasons for the subconscious to block the client's desire to change, and Charles Tebbetts categorized these basic reasons into what he called "The Seven Psychodynamics of a Symptom". They are: authority imprint, current unresolved issue, secondary gain, identifying with someone, inner conflict, self-punishment, and past painful experience. (Charlie originally called the second one "body language" but I changed it to *current unresolved issue* because that is more descriptive.)

The concept is that we may ask the subconscious to reveal (through finger responses) which of the seven psychodynamics are involved in the cause(s) of a problem. Because we must ask such questions as *closed* questions rather than open-ended ones, I emphasize two cautions. First, it is *imperative* that we ask questions regarding all *seven* rather than asking about only one or two of them. Furthermore, this is one time that I strongly urge the therapist to use a *monotone*, in order to minimize the risk or projecting a desired response into the client. Closed questions increase the risk of false perceptions, which lead to false conclusions on the part of client and therapist alike.

Because of the importance of clarity, allow me to repeat what I wrote above in different words. First, by emphasizing that we will ask a series of questions and by using a monotone voice, we reduce the risk of projecting our own expectations into the client.

Before asking the yes/no questions, we must first establish the appropriate finger responses.

3.5.1 Let the client choose the finger responses

Some therapists use involved formulas for determining which finger or thumb to assign for the "yes" or "no" responses. Charlie had a complex formula printed on a handout, complete with diagrams. Long ago I discarded his formula, and recommend against any such formulas. Instead, I ask the client to choose.

Regardless of the therapist's logic for determining the "yes" and "no" fingers, there is an important reason for allowing the client to choose instead: *to avoid confusion*. If a client uses the right index finger for "yes" in one therapist's office, what happens if another therapist assigns that same finger as the negative response? Let's avoid that risk. My words resemble the following:

> I'm going to ask you a series of questions that can be answered "yes" or "no". I would like for you to allow the response to come from your subconscious, or your inner mind.

Note the either/or choice in the above statement, increasing the probability of a subconscious response rather than a conscious one.

> If the answer is "yes", please choose a finger that represents the "Yes" response and indicate by moving it now.

Make a note of it.

> Thank you. If the answer is "N-O", please indicate the negative response by moving that finger or thumb now.

Spell the word "no", and make a note of the response.

> Thank you. If the answer is *either* "I don't know" or "I don't wish to disclose", please choose another finger or thumb and indicate by moving it now.

Also, note that I ask the client to choose a third finger response for "I don't know" or "I don't wish to disclose". Some clients may lie during hypnosis if the desire is strong, and it is not unusual for the subconscious to hide emotional information. Giving this third alternative response increases the probability of obtaining more accurate yes/no responses, further reducing the risk that the therapist might come to false conclusions about the cause of the client's problem.

3.5.2 *Seven important questions (psychodynamics)*

Here are the seven important questions that I ask the client, in order to uncover the subconscious cause(s) of a problem. Remember to ask *all seven* numbered questions *first* before digressing into any "yes" responses provided by the client, as we may often obtain a "yes" response to more than one cause.

Speak the CAPITALIZED words slowly, but without raising your pitch or voice volume, and remember to use a monotone.

> I'm going to ask your subconscious a series of questions related to the CAUSE of the problem … and you may respond with YES or NO, or by moving the "I don't know" finger …

After asking each question, make a note of the response: "yes", "no", or "I don't know [or won't disclose]". Move on immediately to the next question until you ask all seven.

1. Is the cause related to an IMPRINT from an authority figure of past or present?

2. Is the cause related to a current UNRESOLVED ISSUE?

3. Has your subconscious caused that problem because you have something else to GAIN?

4. Are you IDENTIFYING with someone else?

5. Are you feeling an INNER CONFLICT, or two conflicting desires?

6. Was that problem caused by a PAST EVENT?

7. Are you PUNISHING yourself or someone else for something?

After asking all the above questions, we may now explore the YES responses. In some instances, we may need to consider a "don't know" response as a YES response. Here are some tips to help you

YES to an imprint from an authority figure: Find out which authority, and any specifics about the imprint. If unable to get the client to verbalize, use Y/N questions for further exploration (parent, relative, teacher, etc.).

YES to a current unresolved issue: Ask "yes" or "no" whether the issue can be resolved with hypnotherapy. If you receive a "no" response, awaken the client. The unresolved issue *may require a referral to traditional therapy.* Find out what the specific issue is if hypnotherapy is appropriate; otherwise, respect the client's right of privacy.

YES to something else to gain: Continue with Y/N questions … protection? … attention? … sympathy? … manipulate someone? … other? Get specifics.

YES to identifying with someone else: Find out who and why, and what characteristic. If unable to get the client to verbalize, use Y/N questions for further exploration (parent, relative, teacher, friend etc.).

YES to an inner conflict: Parts therapy is indicated.

YES to past event: Regression therapy is indicated.

YES to punishing yourself (self-punishment): Find out why the client indulges in self-punishment. If possible, get the client to verbalize; otherwise, explore with Y/N questions in a monotone voice. Often I choose between parts therapy and regression therapy, depending on the responses and the client's original concern.

In my book, *The Art of Hypnotherapy*, I discuss each of the seven psychodynamics and offer some additional suggestions for potential therapy techniques. In this book devoted to parts therapy, let's consider only those responses that might indicate the use of parts therapy.

The most obvious indicator would be a "yes" response to Question 5 regarding an inner conflict. Frequently I employ parts therapy when the client also responds in the affirmative to *present unresolved issue* (Question 2), *secondary gain* (3), or *self-punishment* (7). Although parts therapy might be appropriate with some people who answer "yes" to the other questions, I normally choose other techniques first. For example, I usually employ regression therapy with the client who answers "yes" to *past event*.

Once I determine that parts therapy may serve my client, my decision to either proceed or wait until the next session depends on two factors: time and explanation. Unless I have at least thirty minutes of session time left, I delay parts therapy until the next session. Even thirty minutes might be insufficient in many cases, depending on the client and the problem. When parts therapy is delayed, I use the remaining time to give some positive suggestions and imagery, and then awaken the client from hypnosis. If time permits me to employ parts therapy the same day, I will proceed only if the client previously received an advance explanation from me regarding parts therapy. Then I'll deepen further before continuing.

In my professional opinion, preparation is almost as important as the parts therapy process itself in order to maximize the potential benefits for the client, so the entire next chapter is devoted to proper preparation. Are you prepared to continue reading?

Chapter 4
Proper Preparation

While I believe in fitting the technique to the client (rather than vice versa), we cannot just wander aimlessly in someone's subconscious without proper preparation. Hypnosis is a journey of mind, and the therapeutic process works best when both therapist and client plan the journey. Advanced planning becomes more important when we are employing parts therapy, because we may encounter a few surprises when we embark on this journey with a client.

Would a hiker walk into the woods without knowing where the trail leads? Even though there may be a few detours along the way, such as a washed-out bridge or a log in the path, the hiker knows where the trail goes. During my backpacking years, I always carried a detailed map of the wilderness area so that I knew exactly where I was at any given time. Before taking my first steps out of the parking lot, I knew which trails and roads were in the area. Additionally, I wanted to know what might be encountered along the way, including any detours from the main path.

The next six chapters reveal my map to successful client-centered parts therapy. When I employ this complex hypnotic therapy technique, I follow a specific path based on the discipline learned years ago from my instructor. My students also learn this same discipline and follow the same path, taking detours only when necessary. This discipline usually leads to excellent results.

Proper preparation begins before the client ever enters hypnosis, and continues during the hypnotic state before we ever call out the first part. Let's begin with the preinduction discussion.

4.1 Explain parts therapy to the client

All of us frequently hear the saying, "An ounce of prevention is worth a pound of cure." When communications are involved, *one minute of communication is worth a month of resolution.*

The above sayings especially apply for clients who experience parts therapy. A woman seeing me for weight management several years ago told me that her first experience with hypnosis frightened her because of her "emerging personalities". Another therapist apparently employed parts therapy without discussing the technique with his client, so she left his office believing that she now had multiple personalities. Fortunately for her, a simple discussion of the technique eased her concerns. It saddened me that six months of anxiety preceded my explanation, which the other therapist should have given to her.

This example emphasizes the importance of providing at least a brief explanation to the client before hypnosis begins. I recommend that we keep the explanation as simple as possible in order to avoid confusing the client. Even now it seems like only a few months ago that Charles Tebbetts wrote "KISS" on the blackboard at his hypnosis school in Edmonds, Washington. One student blurted out, "Keep it simple, stupid!" After a few laughs from the class, Charlie asked if the student was calling him stupid. My instructor used his dry humor to illustrate a very important point regarding the value of speaking in plain language with our clients. He believed that the academic mindset often gave complex explanations for simple concepts, but we should do the reverse when working with clients seeking hypnosis. He told us that esoteric explanations enhance the ego, while simple concepts appeal to the inner child. Because hypnotism directly accesses the inner child, simple explanations obtain better chances of client response.

Although parts therapy is a very complex technique, we can still make the concept easy to understand when discussing it with clients. Usually, the inner child emerges as a part during parts therapy, so I make my explanation both personal and simple, describing my own personality parts in order to help minimize potential client fears. The next paragraph illustrates what I say to clients, which takes less than two minutes:

We all wear different hats for different occasions. For example, I can go to a Friday night movie and think to myself, There is a bargain matinée price on Saturday afternoon. That's the accountant inside my mind reminding me to get the best price. At the same time, my own *inner child* feels that I've worked hard and deserve to have fun when the time is convenient. Under hypnosis, I could easily get into the emotional energy of each part and present conflicting arguments to the hypnotherapist. In an actual past therapy, my inner child had to make a bargain with my *professional self* in order to reach a personal goal. Another way of putting it is that I wear my professional hat here at the office and my inner child hat when it's time to relax and unwind. Many clients wanting to quit smoking have a part that wishes to quit (or they wouldn't see me in the first place), and another part that wants to keep on smoking (or they wouldn't even need my services).

After inviting client questions, I continue with words such as:

> When you attain a relatively deep level of hypnosis, I'll ask that part of your inner mind that wants to attain your goal to simply communicate. Also, I'll ask the other part of your subconscious preventing you from success to speak and be heard. Rather than try to analyze, just go with the flow and get into the feelings that you feel when that part of your mind influences you. My job is to facilitate your own inner dialogue, so that you may attain resolution for inner conflicts regarding quitting smoking [or managing your weight, etc.].

Note my use of the word "try" in the third sentence above. When using hypnosis, never use the word "try" or "trying" unless you do *not* want the client to do what follows that word. Since I do *not* want the client to analyze, I purposely use "try" or "trying" in this instance, and then advise my client to get into his or her feelings.

If you ever have reason to facilitate parts therapy without providing a preinduction explanation, I strongly recommend that you leave some time at the end of the session for discussion so that your client does not leave your office confused about the process. Although I have never personally facilitated parts therapy without advance explanation, I'll concede there could be a rare exception under an unusual circumstance. If and when this ever happens in one of my sessions, I will allow ample time after the session to help my client feel comfortable with the therapeutic process before he/she leaves.

Also, I very rarely use parts therapy on a client's first visit, as I believe the first hypnotic encounter should be enjoyable from start to finish. My two common exceptions are either when I facilitate parts therapy with other therapists, or when helping clients who have enjoyed previous success with hypnotherapy.

41

Let's assume the client accepts the explanation, and is willing to accept his/her role in the parts therapy process. Even after the client enters hypnosis, our preparation has only begun.

4.2 *Hypnotize and deepen appropriately*

Some therapists employ variations of parts therapy with little or no hypnotic trance; but my own experience validates my belief that we can best employ parts therapy when clients are in a deep state of hypnosis. This is why I also consider parts therapy to be *hypnotic inner-conflict resolution*.

Use your induction of choice (assuming the client responds), and deepen appropriately to at least a medium depth level. Just as there are many roads through the states between California and New York, there are many ways to guide a client into deeper hypnotic states. Choose the ones that best fit both therapist and client. If you need to brush up on your deepening techniques, either take a workshop or buy some tapes or books. You might be the best therapist in the world; but, if your client emerges from hypnosis when encountering subconscious resistance, you may lose an important opportunity to help empower that person.

Some variations of parts therapy employ minimal trance states. About two years into my teaching hypnotherapy, a guest presenter talked to my class about voice dialogue. He gave a successful demonstration with one of my students. The similarity to parts therapy motivated me to experience it for myself, not only because of an issue that I needed to overcome, but also because of professional curiosity. During the process, I found it easy to take on the roles of my various parts, but the light trance state allowed too much interference from the analytical side of my brain. The therapist assumed that he facilitated a successful session, but my own inner resolution was only short-lived. After several months I traded sessions with another hypnotherapist competently trained in parts therapy, and finally resolved that inner conflict.

Over the years, various hypnosis associations have given me the opportunity to present parts therapy workshops at their annual conventions. Invariably, I make comments about the importance of deepening to at least a medium level before proceeding into parts therapy, and I often share my experience mentioned above. Other professionals attending my workshops occasionally report similar problems with variations of parts therapy that incorporate only light levels of trance.

While facilitators of voice dialogue can demonstrate many successes, I am not alone in my desire to take my clients into deep hypnotic states while guiding them along the path to inner-conflict resolution. If you want to reduce the risk of analytical resistance, then take your clients to at least a medium hypnotic depth. It is my opinion that facilitators employing voice dialogue might even get better long-term results with more people by using deeper trance states before calling out the parts.

4.3 Establish a safe place

Before commencing the parts therapy process, I guide each client to an ideal peaceful (or safe) place. Even if the client learned this in a previous session, we should reconfirm the safe place and give suggestions for the client to go there immediately when asked to do so. While anchoring the safe place is more important in regression therapy than in parts therapy, I still recommend it because spontaneous regressions sometimes occur. It's better to have a safe place and not need it than it is to need a safe place and not have it.

I normally use open-screen imagery (the client chooses the details), allowing the client to choose his or her ideal, peaceful place. Guided imagery or programmed imagery (the therapist describes the details) would be appropriate only if the client previously described a safe place before entering hypnosis. My suggestions using open-screen imagery are similar to the words below, with emphasis on the words that are capitalized:

> Now, imagine an ideal, peaceful place. Your imagination is your own private rehearsal room of your mind. You can DO ANYTHING you want, or BE ANYWHERE you desire. Just choose a safe, peaceful place, and IMAGINE that you are there now …

> Imagine sights, sounds, and feelings that are SO peaceful, SO serene, and SO relaxing … that it is as though you are becoming a part of the tranquility that you imagine. There is an INNER PEACE just flowing through every part of your being.

The concept conveyed in the sample script above is more important than the exact words. In my opinion, scripts are like training wheels. They serve you while you are learning, but your skills increase when you grow beyond the training wheels. Use any scripts you wish, as long as they follow the discipline of appropriate suggestion structure. Also, make sure that any script serves both you and your clients. Regardless of your choice of words, help the client establish a place inside the imagination that is safe and peaceful from the *client's point of view*.

My sample script uses open-screen imagery rather than guided imagery. During my enthusiastic rookie year as a hypnotherapist, I frequently used guided imagery by asking clients to imagine being in the woods on a pleasant afternoon. One somnambulist suddenly opened his eyes and exclaimed loudly, "*Bugs!* There are too many bugs and mosquitoes in the woods!" He preferred the beach. This mistake resulted in the loss of time and some temporary discomfort for my client. I shared this learning experience with a psychotherapist who also used hypnosis. He told me that he formerly used a beach for a client's safe place until a woman screamed in panic during a session. She was terrified of the ocean.

When working with hospice patients, I make exceptions and use guided imagery, but only after gathering detailed information about the patient's ideal, peaceful place. During hypnosis, I incorporate those details into programmed imagery and guided imagery. For some reason, terminal patients rarely choose more than one peaceful place. However, many clients seeing me for motivation or habit control have more than one safe place, so I normally use open-screen imagery, allowing the client to go wherever he or she chooses.

You may choose your preference: open-screen imagery, or guided imagery. If you choose the latter, make certain to gather sufficient details from your client regarding his or her ideal peaceful place. Remember that one person's safe place might be another person's phobia.

When you perceive the client to be as calm as possible in a safe place, follow with suggestions for the client to return there if and when you suggest it. I ask my client to confirm acceptance of that suggestion by moving a finger that the subconscious chooses as the yes finger. The next step is to either establish or confirm finger responses.

4.4 Establish (or confirm) finger responses

While I rarely resort to ideomotor responding during the parts therapy process itself, my professional experience validates the value of establishing finger responses in advance, or confirming them if established in a previous session. If we wait until encountering a part that refuses to communicate verbally, setting up the ideomotor-response signals could consume time and become a distraction from the therapeutic process. If you are uncertain whether or not to use parts therapy, you may resort to finger-response questioning in order to discover the cause(s) of your client's problem. Chapter 3 contains details of how to establish finger responses (as well as using ideomotor-response questions to discover causes of problems).

Because most parts are willing to communicate verbally, some therapists might consider it a waste of time to establish ideomotor-response signals in advance; but there is another benefit in doing so. Before calling out the first part, I use finger responses to verify hypnotic depth. Read on.

4.5 Verify hypnotic depth

When preparing clients for parts therapy, I use a technique that enables the subconscious to provide feedback that helps to estimate the client's hypnotic depth. Many people consciously underestimate their trance depth (including experienced hypnotherapists), but finger responses often indicate deeper levels than the client might claim verbally.

Let's assume you follow my recommendations presented so far in this chapter. What do you say next? Here is a script that closely resembles what I say:

> Now, imagine a scale of one hundred to the number one. The number one hundred represents being awake but with your eyes closed, while the number one is absolutely as deep as you can go in hypnosis without falling asleep. The number fifty is halfway there. If you are fifty or deeper, please indicate by moving the "yes" finger ...

If yes, continue, if no or "I don't know", then deepen until your client indicates yes. (Note that the above statement is a leading suggestion, designed to lead the client into a state of hypnosis deeper than fifty. Inappropriate leading is when a client responds to leading questions or suggestions that lead him/her into assumptions that could result in fantasy or false memories.)

> Are you forty or deeper?

If yes, continue ... If no, then deepen until client is deeper than forty if you plan on using parts therapy.

> Are you thirty or deeper?

Regardless of the response, ask,

> Are you deep enough to continue into the next part of this session?

If no to the above question, deepen before continuing. If yes to the above question, proceed with parts therapy or the therapy technique of choice. If it is necessary to deepen further, do so and then continue ...

> Are you now 20 or deeper?

If no to the above question, deepen before continuing, and continue doing so until you get a yes. Once you receive a yes reply to the above question, proceed with parts therapy or the therapy technique of choice. If it is necessary to deepen further, do so until you get a yes response and then continue ...

> Thank you. Now that you are deep enough, we will proceed with parts therapy ...

In the scale above, here are my own professional guidelines:

Clients who are unable to get below fifty (after several deepening attempts) will not experience parts therapy with me until another session. Someone who suffers from analysis paralysis will often resist allowing a part to emerge in the first place. Even if we successfully call out the parts in a light level of hypnosis, the risk of conscious interference remains high, minimizing the chances of lasting success. The analytical person in light trance may easily neutralize whatever terms of agreement the parts claim to accept. (As mentioned previously, this opinion comes from my own personal experience as well as the experiences of others reported to me in my workshops.) Once I conclude that a client will not go deep enough for parts therapy during a hypnosis session, I change gears. The client now receives suggestions and imagery, blended with posthypnotic suggestions for attaining a deeper level of hypnosis at the next session.

Some clients who indicate levels between forty and fifty are able to enjoy successful parts therapy, although my preference is to continue with deepening until the level is below forty. The occasional client who responds well between forty and fifty causes me to consider proceeding into parts therapy in this range with some of the people some of the time. However, I always endeavor to deepen below forty first. Again, I prefer more favorable odds.

When responses verify depth levels below forty, my decision revolves around whether the client believes that hypnotic depth is sufficient to continue into the next part of the session. At thirty or below, the client generally accepts suggestions that he/she is now deep enough.

Some clients will ask you to continue deepening until they are too deep to respond verbally, simply because they feel so good going that deep. If a client goes too deep to respond verbally, we may suggest that he/she come up to a level of hypnosis that is still deep, but just high enough to speak verbally. I say words such as, "As I count from one to three, please come up to a level of hypnosis that is still deep, but just light enough for you to speak out loud." I'll have them confirm by saying "Yes" out loud.

Now we are ready to guide the client into the next phase of the journey, which is so important that several chapters are devoted to it. I call it the *eleven-step process*, and this is the *meat* of parts therapy. Let's overview the steps now before exploring them thoroughly.

4.6 Know the eleven-step process

It has been said millions of times that fools rush in where wise men fear to tread. The same can be said for any hypnotist foolish enough to attempt parts therapy without knowing and using all of the vital steps. If you intend to utilize the valuable techniques presented in the chapters to follow, please do both yourself and your clients a favor and walk in the path mapped for you in this book. Memorize the eleven steps so completely that they become automatic whenever you use them. There are some exceptions to my above recommendations, described in the next paragraph.

Some psychologists (and psychotherapists) using hypnosis as an adjunct already obtain numerous client successes using variations of parts therapy that do not incorporate the eleven steps presented in this book. There are many ways to get from Los Angeles to New York, and there may be numerous ways to facilitate inner-conflict resolution. However, unless successful results validate your own way of facilitating parts therapy or one of its variations, I suggest that you give serious consideration to using all of the steps described in the following few chapters.

Before exploring these important steps in depth, I'll list them here, and provide a few closing comments in this chapter. Proper preparation includes at least becoming familiar with all eleven steps in advance until you have them memorized. Feel free to copy the list for your own use with clients as needed.

1. Identify the part.
2. Gain rapport (compliment the part).
3. Call out the part.
4. Thank it for emerging.
5. Discover its purpose.

6. Call out other parts as appropriate.
7. Negotiate and mediate.
8. Ask parts to come to terms of agreement.
9. Confirm and summarize terms of agreement.
10. Give direct suggestion as appropriate (only *after* terms of agreement, but *not* before).
11. Integrate the parts! (The formal parts therapy process is completed.)

4.7 Additional comments

Experienced professionals sometimes approach me during my workshops, claiming that they have never experienced hypnotherapy even though they hypnotize others frequently. While it is not my role to question their reasons or motives, I believe that any competent therapist must be willing to work on his or her own issues when appropriate. We do not have to be perfect in order to be competent with the art of hypnotherapy. As long as we have the integrity to work on our own issues when necessary, we can still be effective. It is my strong opinion that the best salesperson believes in what he or she sells. Hypnotherapists sell empowerment through hypnosis. In order to achieve our ideal effectiveness and conviction with any form of hypnotherapy, I believe that we need to experience it for ourselves.

The late Charles Tebbetts followed the example of Milton Erickson: students learned *by experience*. Likewise, my hypnotherapy students must both give and receive hypnotherapy techniques as a prerequisite for successful completion of my course. Simply hypnotizing others is not enough: my students can more effectively master the art of hypnosis by personally experiencing various hypnotic states. Likewise, I believe that anyone facilitating parts therapy needs to experience it personally. What better way is there to convince a client of the benefits of parts therapy? This experience represents an important part of your advance preparation as a therapist.

Let me also emphasize some additional words of wisdom to the facilitator of this complex but effective hypnotherapy technique. It is vitally important that we remain *nonjudgmental* throughout the entire parts therapy process, even when a part says something that seems ridiculous. Often clients will show a variety of emotions, laughing at themselves, swearing at themselves, and/or expressing surprise at what they say about themselves.

Now let's explore the path to successful client-centered parts therapy.

Chapter 5
The First Four Steps

After properly preparing my client for parts therapy and verifying sufficient hypnotic depth, I move right on into the first four steps. They appear together in one chapter because a skilled therapist may flow through the first three smoothly enough to blend them together almost as one step. The fourth step follows immediately after the part emerges and responds. My students learn the steps by examining each one separately in order to understand what to say, and why.

Although I include scripts where appropriate, you may paraphrase them to your comfort. You should still obtain results with most of your clients if you follow the steps in accordance with the concepts presented in these pages. In addition to the scripts, a sample session is included to further demonstrate the steps. The sample session appears in sans-serif type, and the scripts appear in bold serif type. Rather than asking my students to memorize scripts for the eleven steps, I encourage them to understand the concepts behind each step of the parts therapy process.

5.1 The risk of imagery in parts therapy

Some therapists who enjoy guided imagery and Ericksonian techniques may notice the absence of imagery in most of my scripts. Numerous therapists take the client to an imaginary room with a conference table. Several years ago, I personally experienced parts therapy with a therapist leading me into an imaginary conference room. While that imaginary place was fine for me, similar imagery could push buttons with a client who heard bad news (or got fired) while sitting in a conference room.

Some therapists guide a client to a meadow or some other imaginary place for calling out the parts. Programmed imagery that the client might enjoy, such as a picnic table in the woods, may work well for most clients; but, as we saw in Chapter 4, a forest fantasy could create discomfort or resistance with a client who hates being in the woods.

To avoid the risk of negative reactions, I rarely use guided imagery unless the client initiates it (or requests it in advance). Play it safe and be client-centered.

5.2 Step 1: Identify the part

Most clients with an inner conflict have only two parts involved in the problem. Inner conflicts frequently occur with clients trying to quit smoking, manage weight, or overcome other undesired habits. They may also occur with clients wishing to accomplish personal or professional goals.

The part providing motivation to change (which I call the *motivating part*) causes the client to keep looking for a way to achieve success at the desired goal. The part blocking success (or the *conflicting part*) inhibits the client's best efforts at achieving the goal. We may either call out the motivating part first, *or* we may call out the conflicting part first.

Some therapists start the dialogue with the motivating part. We might logically assume that any subconscious part motivating a client to invest time and money in hypnosis feels comfortable emerging first. This choice often invites considerable dialogue from the motivating part, making it easy for the therapist to start the mediation process. I felt this way during my early years of practice, but discovered a downside to this choice. Sometimes, after first calling out a very vocal motivating part, the conflicting part challenged my patience before I could persuade it to join in the discussion.

My current preference is to identify and call out the conflicting part first. While I occasionally encounter initial reluctance, I'm often able to discover the cause(s) of the inner conflict in less time by working with the conflicting part before the motivating part expresses itself. Sometimes, I make exceptions and call out the motivating part instead, depending on the client and the therapeutic goals. There is no right or wrong choice, because you may still obtain successful results either way. Feel free to choose based on your own preference.

Let's assume my client's name is John (who wants to stop excessive snacking), and I call out the conflicting part first. (We will refer to John throughout the next few chapters.) Here is how I identify the conflicting part …

> **Therapist:** There is a part of you that makes you snack frequently after dinner, and it is doing a very good job. I'm talking to that part of John that causes him to snack frequently.

For a smoker rejecting positive suggestions to quit, we may call out the conflicting part by starting with, "There is a part of you that makes you keep on smoking …" An alternate choice is, "There is a part of you motivating you to quit smoking …"

Before completing the above scripts, let's consider Step 2.

5.3 Step 2: Gain rapport

The primary purpose of the second step is to make each part feel comfortable communicating with the therapist as well as with the client's other part(s). The negotiations for inner-conflict resolution will be much easier if we gain rapport and maintain it throughout the entire session. In my workshops, I explain the importance of rapport with the analogy that parts therapy resembles mediation. Let's consider a metaphor that I use with my students and with therapists attending my parts therapy workshops.

Often during training sessions I single out two students and ask them to pretend they work for different departments in "Company XYZ". Let's call them Linda and Roger. Linda pretends to be the employee wanting Roger's department to change a work procedure, but he wants to maintain status quo. They came to me to resolve their dispute. Linda is like the motivating part and Roger represents the conflicting part. Obviously Linda will probably have a strong desire to come to the mediation table, because she has already demonstrated her motivation to make a change; but what about Roger? He continues working, business as usual, either ignoring Linda or causing her more stress because he believes his way is the right way.

If Linda spills her negative opinions about Roger or his department, how might Roger react if I show any indication of taking Linda's side? My best chance of persuading Roger to talk is to thank him for agreeing to allow me to mediate, compliment him, and make him feel that he may safely communicate his opinions. This metaphor holds true for parts therapy, because we obtain best results by treating each part with the same courtesy and respect as we might use with a separate person.

We start building rapport by complimenting the part and by providing some assurance that it will not be subjected to criticism by the therapist. This especially applies to the conflicting part, because, if it believes the therapist will take sides with the motivating part, the conflicting part might refuse to respond. We must remain neutral throughout the entire parts therapy process, acting like an objective mediator.

By gaining rapport quickly, we increase the chances of effective communication with all parts involved. Conversely, if we sabotage rapport, building it back is much more difficult than gaining and maintaining good rapport from the start. One of my former students lost rapport with a part during parts therapy, and it took him two additional sessions to regain it and get the therapy back on track. (He provided the extra sessions at no charge to compensate her for his mistake.)

I'll return to the metaphor. In my classes, I demonstrate Step 2 by saying, "Roger, thank you for coming to this discussion. You are doing important work for Company XYZ, and probably have good reasons for doing what you are doing. Linda will listen without interrupting, and I will listen ..." The participant in my workshop posing as Roger almost always agrees that he would communicate when asked in this manner. Let's consider an unwise alternative.

His reaction might be very different if I say, "Linda presented a good argument. Why don't you listen to her and apologize for your actions?" When I use this example for the metaphor in workshops, I again ask the student acting in Roger's role what happens to rapport. The response confirms that all rapport is gone, and Roger either refuses to talk or leaves the room.

Now let's get back to John, and notice how building rapport follows immediately after identifying the conflicting part in the first step.

> **Therapist:** There is a part of you that makes you snack frequently after dinner, and it is doing a very good job. I'm talking to that part of John that causes him to snack frequently. You are an important part of John. There is probably a good reason for what you're doing … and you are doing a good job.

Gaining and maintaining rapport is easier when calling out the motivating part; but we still should watch our words closely. If we already called out the conflicting part and it presented a good case to justify its actions, the motivating part might need some persuading to emerge. I'll provide more suggestions regarding rapport with calling out subsequent parts when I cover Step 6 in a later chapter.

5.4 Step 3: Call out the part

Once we identify and compliment that part, it's time to call it out.

> **Therapist:** John is willing to listen, and I am willing to listen. I'm sure that you are doing what you think is right, but another part of John is unhappy, and feels that better communication can enlighten both of you with a few ideas that could make John much happier. If you would like to gain more information and communicate, John is willing to listen to whatever you have to say. When you are willing to communicate, please let us know by saying the words "I am here" or by moving the yes finger.

Charles Tebbetts simply said, "If it's available and wishes to talk, say, 'I am here.' " During my first ten years of practice, about 25 percent of my clients failed to respond when I attempted parts therapy. Although we could speculate a number of different reasons to explain the high resistance rate, I believe in creating more favorable odds whenever possible.

I have two minor updates for Step 3. First, I say "when" rather than "if". (This assumes that the part *will eventually emerge*.) This is a recent update to parts therapy, made in the summer of 2003. The other update (made in the 1990s) involves using an Ericksonian double bind when calling out the part. Instead of giving a part the choice of either emerging or resisting, I give it the *either/or* choice of speaking or communicating by finger response.

Sometimes, we must sell the conflicting part on the idea of emerging and communicating. Any experienced salesperson knows that people are more likely to buy a product when given a choice between two different products (such as color) rather than simply choosing between yes and no. The same holds true for scheduling appointments with people. Giving alternative times is more effective than asking whether or not the person wants the appointment in the first place, because it assumes the person *will agree* to schedule an appointment. Using the word "when" is assumptive, and following that statement with an either/or choice is a simple application of salesmanship. Now let's re-examine what I said above:

> When you are willing to communicate, please let us know by saying the words "I am here" or by moving the yes finger.

The either/or choice is considered an Ericksonian double bind when a client is in hypnosis. Some hypnotists consider the double bind to be a permissive, indirect suggestion. Call it what you wish, but I consider the double bind to be one of the most powerful hypnotic suggestions you can give, because the response ratio is very high. It combines salesmanship with hypnosis. We are selling the inner child, who can be one tough customer. My response ratio has increased by my asking the part to choose between speaking and using finger responses *rather* than to choose between speaking and resisting.

5.5 Combining Steps 1–3

In the sample session with John, note how we may combine the first three steps into several sentences that flow together ...

Therapist: There is a part of you that makes you snack frequently after dinner, and it is doing a very good job. I'm talking to that part of John that causes him to snack frequently. You are an important part of John. There is probably a good reason for what you're doing … and you are doing a good job. John is willing to listen, and I am willing to listen. I'm sure that you are doing what you think is right, but another part of John is unhappy, and feels that better communication can enlighten both of you with a few ideas that could make John much happier. If you would like to gain more information and communicate, John is willing to listen to whatever you have to say. When you are willing to communicate, please let us know by saying the words "I am here" or by moving the yes finger.

What happens if we skip over any of the first three steps? Students of parts therapy often rush through them, forgetting one.

When they fail to identify the part that they wish to call out first, sometimes no part will emerge. At other times an irrelevant part emerges first, but occasionally the right part emerges in spite of the skipped step. The second step is the one most frequently forgotten. Often I witness a student completing a successful parts therapy session even when failing to gain rapport properly. They usually get through the session anyway, but the parts involved are usually more cooperative after building a good rapport. Possible consequences of skipping the third step should be obvious: *the part may not emerge.* Recently, one of my students sat and looked at me quizzically after building rapport because the part would not emerge … until *asked to do so.*

The next chapter section contains additional sample scripts to help you get started with the first three steps. They contain more words than presented earlier in this chapter. Also, rather than use "John" for the client, I use "[client name]" where appropriate. Additionally, the **bold type** makes these scripts stand out in the text. You have my permission to copy the bold-type scripts for your own professional use with clients, but not for distribution to other professionals or students. (If they want these scripts, encourage them to buy this book!)

5.6 Sample scripts

Let's look at two sample scripts: one for calling out the conflicting part, and one for calling out the motivating part. They are revisions of scripts distributed in some of my workshops. Each script combines the first three steps.

5.6.1 Calling out the conflicting part

There is a part of you that makes you snack frequently between meals [makes you keep on smoking, or whatever the client concern is], **and it is doing a very good job. I'm talking to that part of** [client name] **that causes him [her] to snack frequently between meals** [makes you keep on smoking, or whatever the client concern is]. **You are an important part of** [client name], **and there is probably a good reason for what you're doing … and you are doing a good job.** [Client name] **is willing to listen, and I am willing to listen. I'm sure that you are doing what you think is right for** [client name], **but another part of** [client name] **is unhappy, and feels that better communication can enlighten both of you with a few ideas that could make** [client name] **much happier. If you would like to gain more information and communicate,** [client name] **is willing to listen to whatever you have to say. When you are willing to communicate, please let us know by saying the words "I am here" or by moving the yes finger.**

Wait for a response. If there is still no response within about a minute, call out a second time and explain that you are only a mediator. Remind the part that it may speak and be heard! Inner parts are often like children, and a very common complaint among children is that adults *do not listen*! My second attempt contains wording such as:

I am only a mediator, and am telling you what [client name] **told me to say. We are willing to listen to whatever you have to say. Will you please enlighten us, and let me know when you are ready to speak, either by saying "I am here" or by moving the yes finger …**

If there is still no response after two attempts, call out the motivating part first. If the client also fails to allow the motivating part to be called out, there may be *conscious interference*. At your option, you may deepen and try again; or you may call out a third, controlling part. (More information appears in Section 5.9 below.) Unless a part emerges, you may need to switch to another hypnotherapy technique altogether (as I usually do), and attempt parts therapy at the next session.

5.6.2 Calling out the motivating part

There is a part of you motivating you to reach and maintain your ideal weight [motivating you to quit smoking, or whatever the client goal is], **and it is doing a very good job. I'm talking to that part of** [client name] **that wants him [her] to achieve this goal. You are an important part of** [client name]**, and there is probably a good reason for what you're doing ... and you are doing a good job. You motivated** [client name] **to invest time and energy to accomplish this goal. He [she] is willing to listen, and I am willing to listen. I'm sure that you are doing what you think is right for** [client name]**, and there is a good reason why you are doing such a good job. However, another part of** [client name] **wants to prevent you from achieving this goal. Better communication can enlighten both of you with a few ideas that could make** [client name] **much happier. If you would like to gain more information and communicate,** [client name] **is willing to listen to whatever you have to say. When you are willing to communicate, please let us know by saying the words "I am here" or by moving the yes finger.**

Wait for response. If there is no response within about a minute, call out the conflicting part first (if you've not yet done so), using words similar to the appropriate sample script presented earlier in this chapter.

When you become familiar with the above two scripts, vary them as appropriate for each particular client, as well as for your preference. For example, some of my students prefer to ask a part to say "I will" rather than "I am here". One experienced therapist asks a part to agree to communicate by saying "I do", because this response implies further agreements will come later. Others simply ask the part to either say the word "yes" or to move the yes finger. As long as you include the first three steps detailed in this chapter, choose your own words using the script as a guide. Experiment if you wish until you find words that are comfortable to you. Your own comfort (or discomfort) with wording can often be conveyed in a nonverbal manner to clients.

Note that one of my recent students has a strong preference against using a double bind with the first attempt at calling out a part. He is a highly educated, analytical person who feels very uncomfortable being on the receiving end of an either/or choice when talking to a salesperson. From his perspective, a salesperson's double bind is an immediate turnoff. Because of his personal dislike, he will not use a double bind with the first attempt to call out a part. Instead, he waits until the second attempt to call out the part, using the double bind if necessary. Although I prefer my current method, some professionals may prefer to follow the example of my student.

Once the part responds, now what?

5.7 Step 4: Thank it for emerging

This short step can simply be handled with two words: *Thank you*.

If you prefer, you may say, "Thank you for communicating" or "Thank you for being willing to speak and to listen" etc. Although this is the shortest of all the steps, the simple act of expressing thanks helps to maintain rapport. If differing parties participated in mediation for conflict resolution, it would be wise for the mediator to thank those in attendance for their presence, as well as for being willing to discuss their differences. Put the odds in your favor by expressing thanks to each part that emerges. You have nothing to lose by doing so, but your client has something to gain.

5.8 Reviewing Steps 1–4

Now let's put the first four steps together with John, the client wishing to reduce.

> **Therapist:** There is a part of you that makes you snack frequently after dinner, and it is doing a very good job. I'm talking to that part of John that causes him to snack frequently. You are an important part of John, and there is probably a good reason for what you're doing ... and you are doing a good job. John is willing to listen, and I am willing to listen. I'm sure that you are doing what you think is right, but another part of John is unhappy, and feels that better communication can enlighten both of you with a few ideas that could make John much happier. If you would like to gain more information and communicate, John is willing to listen to whatever you have to say. When you are willing to communicate, please let us know by saying the words "I am here" or by moving the yes finger.
>
> **Conflicting part:** I am here.
>
> **Therapist:** Thank you for communicating.

5.9 Possible detours

While guiding the client along the path to successful parts therapy, we occasionally encounter detours blocking the way. Our first potential detour may occur at the third step, and there are four possible blocks:

- the conflicting part won't speak until the motivating part speaks first (or vice versa);
- neither of the parts in conflict will speak unless a third, controlling part allows it;
- the client will not respond to parts therapy;
- the part will only provide finger responses.

The first possible block is the most common, and the easiest to get around. The second one may take trial and error combined with patience. The third one may prevent parts therapy altogether, but could be mistaken for the second detour. The fourth detour is the most challenging. My modus operandi for each detour follows …

If a part fails to emerge when first called out, we do not yet know whether a detour even exists, much less which of the above it might be. After calling out the conflicting part, I wait up to about a minute for the response before calling it out again. One minute passes very slowly when your client is silent, so watch your watch. If the second request fails to obtain a response, I call out the motivating part first instead of the conflicting part (or vice versa). A response from the other part obviously indicates getting past the first detour successfully.

If neither of the parts in conflict emerges after two attempts apiece, my final attempt is to find out whether there is a controlling part. Although this second potential detour is rare, here is what I ask:

> Is there any other part that wishes to speak first? If so, either say the words "I am here" or move the yes finger.

If there is no response to the above question, we may assume that we have the third detour described above. In this case, I'll usually abort parts therapy for that session. I simply give some suggestions and imagery, along with posthypnotic suggestions for a more successful session next time. After awakening the client, I discuss parts therapy further with him or her so that he or she may feel more comfortable with the technique at the next visit. Although this happens far less frequently now than in my first ten years of practice, some clients still try to overanalyze the hypnotic process and resist parts therapy for one reason or another. If there is no response to parts therapy the following week, I will use other hypnotherapy techniques instead.

When I receive an affirmative response to calling out a third part, I proceed with Steps 4 and 5. Sometimes this "third" part is actually one of the first two parts originally called out, which will become apparent while proceeding through Step 5 (described in the next chapter). However, if this part seems to be a controlling part or a neutral part, I ask an important question:

What must I do to call out the other parts of [client name]?

Several years ago a controlling part identified itself as Secretary. She responded to the above question by telling me somewhat authoritatively, "I control all the file folders for Jane's parts, and you must ask me to open the filing cabinet and give you the folder for each part you wish to talk to." Before going any further, I asked Secretary to provide the files for that part of Jane that caused her to smoke, as well as the part motivating her to quit smoking. She informed me that the requested files would be placed on the table in the conference room, so that each part could enter the room and talk to me. The remainder of that parts therapy session incorporated the conference room imagery provided by my client.

On another occasion, a part emerged that identified itself as the Inner Adviser, who had to approve of any other part speaking with me. While no imagery was involved here, the Inner Adviser silently observed the rest of the session, speaking again only after the other parts reached terms of agreement. The Inner Adviser then advised each part to honor its promises.

Another hypnotherapist once told me that he always calls out a controlling part before ever calling out the two parts in conflict. My professional experience indicates that to be an unnecessary step with most of the people most of the time, so I call out only the parts that need to be involved in the parts therapy process instead. Usually only the conflicting and motivating parts will emerge, making the therapy easier for both client and therapist alike.

My comments on handling the fourth detour occur in the last section of Chapter 6.

Now let's move on and examine Step 5, which is so important that I devoted an entire chapter to this step in order to present it thoroughly.

Chapter 6
The Important Fifth Step
Discover Its Purpose

Once I thank the part for emerging, I move right on to the important fifth step. Discovering the part's purpose can take anywhere from one minute to over twenty minutes, varying from client to client. The best way to discover the primary purpose of a part is to simply ask; but my first question is to ask the part about its name or title.

6.1 Why should a part choose a name or title?

Asking this question often results in clues that may help the therapist discover the core cause quickly, because the primary purpose of a part is often the title that will be chosen. This may reduce the number of additional questions required to obtain accurate and thorough information about the part's purpose. My question is simple, immediately following Step 4: "What name or title do you wish to be called?"

I make a note of it. If the emerging part initially responded with a finger movement rather than verbally, I still ask the same question about its name or title. Often this question elicits a verbal reply even after an initial ideomotor response. (You will find suggestions in the last section of this chapter for handling the rare part that insists on giving finger responses rather than verbal replies.) Remember that sometimes the motivating part may emerge first even when we attempt to call out the conflicting part first, or vice versa. Let's resume our sample therapy session with John.

Therapist: What name or title do you wish to be called?

Conflicting part: I'm Happy.

Note the clue regarding the part's purpose is evident in the name it chose. The conflicting part for smokers will often give titles or names such as Happy, Silly, Smokey, The Rebel, Freedom, Billy (inner child), Jenny, or other proper names that may or may not provide insight. Dieters often have a conflicting part that gives titles such as Happy, Silly, Eater, Playful, Pleasure, Billy (inner child) etc. Motivating parts provide names such as Healthy, Motivator, Success, William (inner adult), Jennifer etc.

Generally, better clues are provided with titles than in names, with one common exception. An adult version of a name, such as Robert or Kathleen, usually indicates a motivating part. A child version of a name, such as Johnny or Cathy, usually indicates that we are speaking with the inner child. Exceptions sometimes occur, so never assume.

One published hypnotherapist (whom I will not name here) criticized in print the practice of allowing a part to have a name or title, claiming that the benefit is questionable. That particular hypnosis teacher has clients put the energy of the two conflicting parts into each hand, with kinesthetic imagery. While such a technique might get results, this instructor's book states that a name or title creates a stronger identity that enhances the separateness from the main personality. I'll concede that the author's written statement might sometimes be temporarily true during portions of the parts therapy process, but I find this separateness often keeps the conscious mind from analyzing the process too soon. I do not consider that instructor's concern to be a problem as long as the therapist follows all the proper steps of parts therapy presented in my classroom, including integration when terms of agreement are confirmed. My opinion is validated by the many successes of my own students, as well as the late Charles Tebbetts, who always asked a part to provide a name or title when he demonstrated parts therapy in his classroom. I reject the criticism that my methods are questionable when they produce good results, and will continue to practice and teach what has worked for my clients since 1983. (That being said, I still update my methods when valid reasons indicate the need to do so.)

In addition to discovering clues about a part's primary purpose, there is another benefit in asking a part to choose a name or title. Facilitating the client's inner dialogue is much easier when the therapist knows the name or title of each emerging part, especially if three or more parts participate in the dialogue.

John's motivating part called itself Success, which also summarized its job function. (More about Success will come later.)

6.2 Ask the "W" questions

Even when the name or title indicates a part's purpose, Step 5 is not a short step. Additional information is almost always necessary regarding a part's primary purpose, as well as how the part influences the client. I teach my students to simply ask the "W" questions: *what, when, where, who, why,* and *how.* (Although I admit that it's a stretch, "how" ends in "w" so we can still find a logic in calling it one of the "W" questions.)

I want to know *what* the part's primary purpose is and *how* that part accomplishes that purpose. Depending on the response to the first two questions, I may need to know *when* and *why* a part first started doing its current job. The answers to these questions are often quite enlightening to both client and therapist alike. When necessary, I continue asking questions to gather any additional information pertinent to moving the client closer to resolution. When asking these additional questions, it's important to avoid inappropriate leading. (In other words, avoid asking yes/no questions.)

Throughout this process, endeavor to maintain rapport by asking politely rather than appearing like an attorney interrogating a witness in court. Sometimes, I've heard students asking one question after another, in rapid fire, without any pauses—until the part starts reacting defensively to the questions. Once you ask a question, *listen* to the response and make notes. Writing notes will generally force the therapist to listen well, and to pause between questions. Also, parts frequently pause longer than a person in normal conversation does, so I normally wait several seconds before continuing. If I accidentally interrupt a part, I stop talking and continue listening. Any deliberate interruption should be rare.

Now let's explore each of the "W" questions that may be asked during Step 5, beginning with the one that I always ask first after a part tells me its name or title. I'll continue with John's sample session.

6.2.1 What ...?

Most of the time the part will respond to a direct question about its primary purpose, especially when asked in a straightforward manner. Here are my usual words:

Therapist: Hi, Happy! What job do you do for John?

Happy: I make him do things that make him happy.

Again, you may change the wording if you wish, but keep the question simple. One of my former students asks, "What is your job function for John?" If preferred, you could ask, "What is your primary purpose for John?" Then make a note of the response.

If the part has already given you a probable purpose in the title, such as Happy, then it may be acceptable to ask a leading question (under those circumstances only). In such a case, you could ask, "Is it your job to keep John happy?"

When the part discloses its job, I often continue with another similar question: "What else do you do for John?" This additional open-ended question can often be helpful in obtaining important insight.

Responses I have heard from the conflicting part are:

- *I make John happy.*
- *I want Linda to enjoy the freedom to smoke [or eat] when she wants.*
- *I make Kevin take time to play or have fun, and smoking [or snacking] is fun.*
- *I protect Martha from ... [getting into a relationship etc.]*
- *I help Tom to be like ... [relative, celebrity, sports hero or other mentor].*
- *I don't have to do what my parents tell me any more.*
- *I punish Bob when he gets sidetracked.*

- *I protect Judy's right to enjoy life.*
- *Nobody is going to tell me to quit smoking [or quit snacking etc.].*
- *I'm FREE, and my … [church, employer etc.] doesn't have the right to tell me what to do.*
- *I make sure Susie continues to belong to the Smoker's Minority.*

Typical responses from the motivating part are:

- *My job is to help Diane stay healthy.*
- *I help Roger make good decisions.*
- *I motivate Karen to be a good person.*
- *I help Bob to succeed in life.*
- *I keep Linda on the right path.*
- *My job is to help Ray achieve his full potential.*
- *I help Marlene be the best she can be.*
- *My job is to help Tim achieve his goals.*
- *I help Judy do what God wants her to do.*
- *I remind David that it's time to grow up.*

The above responses come in many different words, but they usually relate to the inner conflict between achieving a goal and refusing to pay the price of achievement. Usually, the motivating part wants the client to overcome an undesired habit in order to be a better person (healthier, better looking, having a better self-image, having personal success etc.). Conversely, the conflicting part normally keeps the person stuck in the old habit for one (or more) of a number of varied reasons: temporary enjoyment, rebellion, self-punishment, present unresolved issue, personal identity, identification with a mentor, secondary gain (such as protection from relationships), and occasionally some other strange reason.

On occasion the conflicting part provides a very constructive job function or primary purpose that seems unrelated to the habit the client wants to overcome. One common example I've encountered many times over the years is an inner child that wants the client to take time to play because he/she is a workaholic (an example of *present unresolved issue*). Further questioning often reveals that the inner child causes a habit to get out of control as a way of getting the client's attention so that the client will make some other important changes of habit or lifestyle.

While this first "W" question is the most important one to ask regarding a part's primary purpose, we normally need to know more than is initially disclosed. However, sometimes a part becomes so talkative that all we need do is listen and take notes while it answers all the remaining "W" questions without any further prompting. The other questions are listed according to the importance that I give them in this step. Although I usually ask them in this order, I remain flexible to exceptions.

6.2.2 How ...?

My own professional experience indicates a frequent value in knowing *how* a part accomplishes its job. Unless the part has already disclosed "how" it performs its purpose, I almost always ask. Again, I keep my words simple: "How do you do that?" If desired, we may repeat the part's response after asking the "what" question. For example, John's conflicting part confirmed that its job was to make John happy. My next question was, "*How* do you make John happy?"

The responses often parallel those given to the first question, with added clarification. Here are four typical responses:

- *I make him [John] happy at night because he likes the taste of food.*
- *I give Linda smoking urges whenever people tell her to quit.*
- *I make Bob happy by giving him smoking urges and making him respond to them.*
- *I protect Mary from a bad relationship by making her so fat that most men wouldn't want her.*

There may be various other responses, which may provide important information to both therapist and client in the steps that follow. Again, be certain to make notes, as they often prove to be quite valuable later in the session.

When such information is obtained, it often makes it easier to obtain terms of agreement; but let me emphasize a word of caution mentioned earlier in this chapter. To avoid being perceived as an interrogator, we should limit the number of questions we ask. If we put the conflicting part on the defensive, the loss of rapport can make the rest of the parts therapy more difficult for both client and therapist alike. There is an old saying: "You can catch more flies with honey than with vinegar." The metaphoric lesson in that saying is that diplomacy and respect will go much farther than an authoritative approach when we communicate with a client's subconscious part.

If the part provides sufficient information in the first two "W" questions, I often proceed directly into Step 6 and then come back to the remaining questions in this step later if necessary. However, if the information obtained from the first two questions is minimal, then I continue with more questions before calling out any other part. Also note that answers to the first two questions above are normally sufficient when talking with a third part (or a controlling part) not in conflict with either of the first two parts.

6.2.3 Why ...?

When necessary, I not only ask the part *why* it does its job: I sometimes inquire about the motive behind the motive. Knowing *why* a conflicting part wants my client to stay in the current behavior pattern often provides valuable insight. This information might be as important as learning why the part accomplishes its primary purpose. The answers will sometimes differ (in which case I list both of them).

For example, one of my overweight clients had a conflicting part that called itself Silly, and its purpose was to give Donna pleasure. Silly quickly told me *how* she gave pleasure: "By making Donna give in to snacking urges." The obvious response to why Silly did her job was because everyone needs to have some pleasure in life, so there was no need to ask that question. Instead, I continued with, "Why do you make Donna get her pleasure through snacking?" The response to that second question was very enlightening. Silly went on to complain about how life is nothing but work, and that all Donna wanted to do was be a good mother and wife, a perfect professional, and a good Christian, who never took time for personal pleasure. We also will find the occasional client who indulges in excessive pleasure and has a conflicting part that punishes the client for it.

Some typical responses gathered from the conflicting part over the years are listed below. While the wording might vary, they convey information commonly disclosed. (They often resemble responses to the "what" question.) Those with an asterisk(*) frequently require additional exploratory questions, such as obtaining the motive behind the motive. For example, a response indicating self-punishment requires that we ask why the part is punishing our client etc.

- *I'm punishing Jim for not being good.*
- *Everyone needs to have fun.*
- *I don't have to do what my parents tell me anymore.*
- *Because of what Larry did (or does).*
- *Because it feels good.*
- Martha needs to have freedom of choice, and people keep trying to take her choice away.
- I'm tired of society discriminating against fat people.
- I'm tired of the do-gooders pressuring everyone to quit smoking.
- *Simply because it's fun.*
- Mark works too hard, so I make sure he does something that gives him pleasure.
- Because my father (or mother) smokes.
- Everyone in my family is overweight.
- Mary wants life to be all work and no play.
- *Because of what Mommy (or another person) did. (Ask "what" and "when" with this response, and prepare for a possible spontaneous regression.)
- *Because of what Mommy (or another person) is doing. (Ask "what" the other person is doing. The response may require that you refer the client to another professional unless you are qualified to deal with the issue that emerges. See Section 6.3 below.)
- *I want to get John's attention because he needs to … (The part may describe some behavior pattern of the client that is not previously known to the therapist.)

Let me comment on the last response. When a part gives me a response similar to the last one shown above, I say, "Well, you got John's attention, and he is willing to listen. Please tell him exactly what you want him to do, and how you want him to do it." After making a note of the response, I'll then thank the conflicting part for communicating, and move right on to Step 6. (See my comments in the next chapter regarding this next step.)

When talking with the motivating part, I usually ask that part to explain why the client should achieve the desired goal (unless that information was previously disclosed). Additional explorations are not needed as frequently as when communicating with the conflicting part. Now let's consider some typical responses from the motivating part when I do ask the "why" question:

- *I want John to stay healthy.*
- *Donna will have more energy if she quits smoking [or loses weight].*
- *Joe needs to look good to attract the right woman into his life.*
- *Ed needs to look good in order to make his wife happier.*
- *Cindy needs a good personal [and/or professional] image.*
- *Bob needs to be all he can be.*
- *This is just something that Don needs to do for himself.*

If I get this last response, I will usually ask why it is important for Don to do this for himself. Additional clarification might be appropriate, such as, "How do you expect Don to do this?" Numerous other responses have emerged over the years besides the above samples.

6.2.4 When …?

Sometimes, I ask, "When did you first take on this job?" The responses vary, and occasionally may result in a spontaneous regression. When this occurs, we may facilitate the regression and endeavor to discover and release the core cause. I continue to ask the "W" questions during a spontaneous regression, tailoring them to the information disclosed by the part. Abreactions with a part are often (but not always) milder than when regression therapy is facilitated outside of parts therapy. Once the regression is completed, we must remember to return to parts therapy and resume either with this same step or the next one.

6.2.5 Who …?

This question is exploratory when further clarification is needed after asking previous questions. I might ask "who" if earlier responses indicate the need to know who else is (or was) involved with causing or contributing to a part's purpose. Although normally asked during a spontaneous regression, this question is frequently irrelevant during parts therapy without regressions.

6.2.6 Where …?

This question is also optional, unless needed for further clarification of responses given previously. Frequently, I skip this question as well except during a spontaneous regression.

6.2.7 John's sample session

My sample session with John reveals how much information I might gather in a typical session that flows smoothly through Step 5.

Therapist: What name or title do you wish to be called?

Conflicting part: I'm Happy.

Therapist: Hi, Happy! What job do you do for John?

Happy: I make him do things that make him happy.

Therapist: I see. How do you make John happy?

Happy: Well, I make him snack at night because he likes the taste of food.

Therapist: Is there anything else you do to make him happy?

Happy: No. He gets pleasure when I tantalize his taste buds.

Therapist: Why do you feel that tantalizing his taste buds is necessary in order to keep him happy?

Happy: Well, he never takes time to do anything else that makes him happy, and he deserves some happiness in life. He only seems to have time for the three "Ws".

Therapist: What are the three "Ws"?

Happy: Work, work, work!

Therapist: Would you please explain further?

Happy: Well, John is proud of his success—but he works too hard. He is so busy being a good worker, a good father, a good husband, and a good Christian that he never takes time to *enjoy* his success. What good is working to be successful if you can't take time to enjoy some of it yourself?

Therapist: Thank you for communicating. You provided some very important information. Would you be willing to listen now while I call out another part of John?

Happy: Yes.

Therapist: Thank you.

Note my last comments above from the continuing sample session with John. Upon obtaining sufficient information to call out the motivating part, I thanked Happy for communicating. Also, *I asked him to listen* while I called out another part. Before moving on, however, there are some concerns that I wish to explore.

6.3 Possible detours

Occasionally, the conflicting part will reveal a cause that requires the client to make a conscious decision to resolve. Here are two examples that happened in my office.

Years ago a woman seeing me for weight reduction had a conflicting part say, "I'm not letting her get rid of this weight until that male chauvinist pig she's married to overcomes his bias against fat women." There was no compromise. The conflicting part revealed the cause as an external, ongoing one, and my client had no control over her husband's attitude. I awakened her out of hypnosis after giving her suggestions that she would deal with her weight in the time and manner that were appropriate for her highest and best good. Although I suggested marriage counseling, she said that her husband's attitude was his problem now instead of hers. Six months later she called me and said, "I hope you didn't consider me a failure when I saw you. Since I'm only about thirty pounds over-weight, I have decided that I like who I am. My husband can love me for who I am rather than how my body looks. I wish I would have seen you five years ago and five thousand dollars ago!"

Another client saw me for an inner conflict regarding weight man-agement. When I called out what I believed was his conflicting part, it said, "My job is to help Jim resolve problems instead of running away from them. He knows which problem he is running away from, and I caused him to put on this weight in order to get his attention that he needs to confront that issue." When I called out the other part, it was Jim's conscious mind, who then said that nothing more could be done in hypnosis. At the conscious level, he told me that it was a total surprise to find out that the cause of his weight was related to his unresolved family problem. He said that he knew what had to be done, and would see a counselor for some advice before making a difficult decision. To this day I don't know what Jim's particular issue was, or whether it was related to family or job. He left my office telling me that he discovered some important information from his inner mind, but he never saw me again.

A more serious detour occurs when it becomes apparent that the cause is something requiring other professional help. For example, on rare occasions the cause of a client's inner conflict may be the result of living in an abusive relationship. Unless you have experi-ence with abuse counseling, choose your words carefully. I refer these people to other professional help.

6.4 Avoid inappropriate leading

Once the part starts disclosing the requested information, we need to keep additional questions open-ended as well. Let's suppose a part smokes because of John's parents. It would be *inappropriate leading* to ask, "Are you punishing John for disobeying his parents when he started smoking?" Instead, ask something such as, "How do John's parents influence the job you are doing for him?" During my first few years of teaching hypnotherapy, some overeager students made assumptions and started assuming what the responses would be by asking yes/no questions. Although far more risky in regression therapy, inappropriate leading could take us down the wrong path during parts therapy as well.

Occasionally, we might call out the conflicting part, only to discover the motivating part emerging first (or vice versa). For example, one student who took my class over a decade ago was working with another student regarding her weight. When he attempted to call out the conflicting part first, it gave itself the title of Happy. Then he asked, "Do you make Karen happy by making her eat too many snacks?" The part quickly responded by informing him that Karen would be happier if she controlled her eating habits and became more slender. Although he assumed that the conflicting part emerged first, the motivating part emerged instead. No damage was done, but we can easily see the wisdom in two important words: *never assume*.

An office supervisor saw me who had a conflicting part called Success. After confirming that its job was to make Tom successful, I understandably assumed that the motivating part emerged first. Fortunately, I did not make that assumption known. Instead, I asked *how* it accomplished its job and got a confusing answer: "It's important for Tom to succeed at work, so I make him overweight." After asking *why* Success made Tom gain weight, that part went on to explain that it was to protect Tom from an attractive subordinate who had previously asked him out. (Over the years, several clients have had parts reveal a similar cause for being overweight: protection from affairs.) She liked slender men, so the part that motivated Tom to be successful also caused him to gain enough weight to protect him from an affair in the workplace. The part motivating him to reduce called itself Balance, and later persuaded him simply to say a polite no to her advances.

Because we are human, it is easy to make assumptions, as I almost did in the above example; but we need to do our best to avoid projecting any of those assumptions into the therapy session. Had I projected my assumption into the session with Tom, who knows what might have happened? At best, time (and the client's money) would have been wasted walking into an unnecessary detour.

One of the worst examples of inappropriate leading I ever witnessed occurred at a workshop. The facilitator called out a conflicting part causing a woman to be overweight, and then commanded, "If you are an influencing or attaching entity, then move the yes finger." When there was no immediate response, he spoke loudly with even more emphasis: "If you have either an attaching or influencing entity, move the yes finger." Needless to say, I was not surprised when the woman volunteer moved her yes finger. After her embarrassment motivated her to avoid eating lunch with the rest of us, I facilitated a private session with her to undo the damage done by the unnecessary guilt laid upon her in front of several dozen of her peers.

On rare occasions, a part that is not even involved in the client's inner conflict may emerge when you call out the first part. If so, deal with what emerges. Do not assume that you can get that part to remain quiet while you call out the two parts in conflict first. A woman seeing me for weight reduction several years ago had a part that called itself Guard, who had to inspect my office and make sure it was safe. Since I was still uncertain whether or not this was the conflicting part, I proceeded through Step 5 and discovered that Guard's job was to protect both my client and her parts. He then escorted each participating part into the discussion area before I could ask any questions. What might have happened during the therapy process if I had assumed Guard was the conflicting part instead of a controlling part?

6.5 Sample scripts

It is difficult to provide scripts for all the situations that may be encountered during many of the steps of parts therapy, and this is especially true of Step 5. However, I'll provide some that may get you going. As with other scripts, paraphrase them to your liking.

Just remember to ask open-ended questions. Then be sure to listen to your client and take good notes.

What job do you do for [client name]**?**

What is your primary purpose?

How do you do that?

How do you accomplish that?

How do you [make client happy etc.]**?**

Why do you need to do that?

Why do you [cause client to eat, smoke etc.]**?**

When did you first take on this job?

Who told you that you needed to do that?

Where did that happen?

Ask additional "W" questions as appropriate, depending on the responses to the above questions. Be sure to give the part an opportunity to listen to the other part(s) after it provides sufficient information, preferably before if gets too defensive.

Once we obtain sufficient information, it's time to call out the other part. Before doing so, however, I say something that maintains rapport with the first part while making the next part feel safe before it is ever called out. My words resemble the following:

Thank you for sharing. You provided some important information. Are you willing to listen now while I call out another part of [client name]**?**

If there is a delay in responding, continue with,

I'll give you an opportunity to respond after that other part speaks.

Once I receive a yes response, it's time to call out another part—or to allow the other part to respond again if it was called out earlier in the session. Also note: by getting the first part to agree to listen, calling out the other part becomes much easier, especially if the motivating part emerged first and the conflicting part has yet to speak. Before moving on to that step, however, I wish to include two more sections in this chapter.

6.6 *Important advice from Charles Tebbetts*

The advice that Charles Tebbetts gave more often than any other is a sentence with only four words: "Deal with what emerges." The astute reader will probably notice this same advice appearing elsewhere in this book more than once.

As is obvious by now, sometimes we might call out the conflicting part first, and the motivating part emerges (or vice versa). I simply deal with it and go with the flow, rather than insist that the client's parts follow my own plans. Occasionally, a neutral part emerges first. At times the core cause may be a total surprise to both client and therapist alike, indicating a different destination than the one originally planned. For example, a smoker wishing to quit might end up smoking occasionally rather than quitting totally; or an overweight person may discover something more important that he or she needs to change first before dealing with being overweight.

Indeed, while the above advice remains as important today, I wish to share some other important words of wisdom learned both from my mentor and from the school of experience.

Charlie taught us to always endeavor to put ourselves in the place of a client, realizing that we might act (or react) the same way if we were in that person's shoes with his/her same life experiences. With that in mind, he encouraged us never to criticize a part for doing its job. Occasionally, a part will claim a job or purpose that is totally bizarre, such as something destructive. Rather than try to destroy a destructive part or criticize it, I still proceed through the

"W" questions as usual. Later on in the session the potentially destructive part (or disowned part) usually takes on a new job, either by choice or by request from another part. This is more easily accomplished with courtesy than with criticism.

I'll take this one step farther. When we are facilitating parts therapy, we should treat each part as though it is a separate person feeling justified in fulfilling its purpose for the client. Although conflicting parts are often aspects of the inner child, one common complaint among children is that *adults don't listen* to them. Listening is crucial throughout the parts therapy process, and courtesy helps to maintain rapport. Be especially careful when you have an inner child part that gets argumentative or whines about another part (or the person).

Some students have debated my above opinion over the years, but I have yet to witness a *parts* therapy session go sour because of treating a *part* with too much diplomacy and objectivity while asking about its purpose. An ounce of courtesy goes much farther than a pound of criticism when one is dealing with an argumentative part. Often I can help it calm down by inviting it to vent until everything is expressed—and then I feel totally justified asking it to listen while I call out the other part.

Let's return to the metaphor of Roger and Linda. Remember that Roger is the conflicting employee (or *part*) and Linda is the motivating employee (or *part*) of Company XYZ. If I ask Roger about his purpose and then criticize Linda for wanting him to change, what happens to my rapport with Linda? In my professional opinion, we can do a far better job of mediating objectively by putting ourselves in the place of each part (rather than just the conscious integrated client). After listening to each part, and giving each part the opportunity to communicate to its fullest desire regarding the primary purpose, we will be better able to effectively continue with the next important step in the therapeutic process.

Before moving on to that step, however, we need to consider how to handle an occasional obstacle that may sharpen our therapy skills.

6.7 Parts that use finger responses

My own ultimate challenge occurs when a part refuses to respond verbally. When a part emerges with a finger response instead of replying verbally, I ask yes/no questions and endeavor to do so in a way that reduces the risk of leading.

My first response remains the same: "Thank you. What name or title may I call you?"

Often this question results in a verbal response, and I proceed as described in the previous pages. If the part remains silent, I continue in a monotone with words such as:

You are either the part that causes [client name] **to** [smoke, overeat etc.]**, or you are the part that motivates him to change, or another part altogether. Please respond with the yes or no finger as I ask you which part you are …**

Are you the part that wants [client name] **to continue** [smoking, overeating etc.]**?** If the reply is no, then continue …

Are you the part that motivates [client name] **to** [quit smoking, reduce etc.]**?** If the reply is NO, then continue …

Are you another part altogether?

One of these three questions almost always results in a yes reply. If not, I ask them again with a little more emphasis (unlike typical ideomotor-response questioning).

If the yes response comes from the conflicting part, I proceed through the same questions that you will find in Section 3.5 in Chapter 3, "Psychodynamics and ideomotor responding" (see the sample questions in Chapter 3). Again, I revert to a monotone voice throughout this form of questioning in order to minimize the risk of inappropriate leading. Once I have completed the basic questions regarding the psychodynamics, I ask a very important question: "Are you willing to discuss this verbally?" If the response is yes, the rest of the parts therapy process becomes much easier. Sometimes, it may take a little coaxing; but, if you can make the conflicting part feel that it can safely communicate and be heard, the therapy will be easier for both you and your client. However, if the response is still no (this happens rarely), then I will ask if another part can communicate verbally on behalf of the part that won't speak, or if another part will act as an interpreter. Though it is cumbersome, I prefer this method of communication to continued finger-response questions.

If the motivating part is the one that replies only by finger response, my work is cut out for me (especially if the conflicting part has already spoken its peace). Although I can count on my hand the number of times I've encountered this situation over the years, my best advice is to deal with what emerges and make the part feel safe in communicating verbally. Do your best to persuade the part to speak verbally, and be prepared to call out a third part if necessary.

On those occasions where a part replying with finger-response answers no to the first two questions and yes to the third question, further exploration frequently reveals it to be the conflicting part. Perhaps the resistance to change emerged with finger responses rather than verbal communication in these cases.

In spite of the above advice, one of the most challenging parts therapy sessions I ever facilitated took place when both the conflicting and motivating parts responded only with finger responses. Although this happened only once to me in twenty years, the session was successful. I asked each part to communicate its primary purpose to both the conscious mind and the other part involved. Then, when calling out the other part, I asked, "Are you aware of the other part's primary purpose and how that purpose is accomplished?" From here, I asked each part to let the other part know what it desired, and what it would do in exchange—and to confirm this by moving the yes finger. The client never even told me what agreements were made between the conflicting and motivating parts, but apparently she achieved her desired goal. She taught me that we could employ a form of indirect parts therapy and still get results! Since this unusual case, I have often employed a variation of this indirect parts therapy by calling out only one part: a client's *innermost wisdom*. This will be explained in Chapter 13.

For now, let's assume the first part provided sufficient information, and it's time to call out another part. When concluding Step 5, remember to ask the part to *listen* while you call out another part.

Chapter 7
Let the Mediation Begin

Once we call out the conflicting part, we must call out the motivating part (or vice versa) before any negotiations or mediation can take place. That being said, I set the table for mediation early in Step 6.

7.1 Step 6: Call out other parts as appropriate

This step is more complex than the fifth one because it usually incorporates repeating the first five steps at least once. The procedure varies, depending on which part emerged first (the conflicting part or the motivating part). We will explore both possibilities in this chapter section, followed by two additional possible situations. Since I encourage my students to call out the conflicting part first, the motivating part will be the one most commonly called when reaching Step 6 for the first time.

7.1.1 Calling out the motivating part

Once the conflicting part expresses its primary purpose to the satisfaction of the part and therapist alike, we may now call out the motivating part. Before doing so, however, remember to thank the conflicting part for communicating, and ask it to *listen* while other parts speak. Then, we may repeat Steps 1 through 4 as explained earlier, using similar scripts. Although I abbreviate Step 5 the second time around, I still want to verify the motivating part's purpose in order to be sure that the correct part emerges, as another part may occasionally emerge instead.

Let's return to my sample session with John. His conflicting part was Happy; and now it's time for me to call out the motivating part.

Therapist: ... and now, I'd like to talk to that part of John that motivates him to reach his ideal weight and control his eating habits. You are an important part of John, and there is probably a good reason for what you're doing ... and you motivated him to invest his time and money to participate in these sessions, so you are doing a good job. Happy is willing to listen, and I'm willing to listen. When you are ready to speak, please say the words "I am here" or move the yes finger.

Motivating part: I am here.

Therapist: Thank you for communicating. What name or title should I call you?

Motivating part: I'm Success.

Therapist: Hi, Success! What job do you do for John?

Success: I motivate him to be all he can be.

Therapist: [pause ... I'm listening in case Success continues.]

Success: John sets good goals, and I help him to achieve them. He is a good person, and I motivate him to stay that way.

Therapist: That's a very important job, but did you hear what Happy said?

Success: Yes.

Note that my only question regarding Step 5 was, "What job do you do for John?" After obtaining this information, I moved right on to a rare leading question: "... but did you hear what Happy said?" This is one of those occasions when it is appropriate to lead, because we are not implanting our own conclusions about the therapy into the client. However, since it was important for Happy to hear what Success said, such a question is both appropriate and necessary.

Invariably, I get a yes response to that leading question (up to the writing of this book). What I say next sets the table for the rest of the parts therapy steps.

Therapist: Thank you for listening to Happy. Happy has agreed to listen to you now, so how do you respond to what Happy said?

Success: John gets great satisfaction at being successful in business, and in having a good marriage and stable family. He always accomplishes whatever he puts his mind to do, because I'm always here to help him; but we can't seem to get that extra weight to go away because of Happy. Yet Happy says his job is to make John happy, and I know that John would be happier if he could get rid of thirty pounds.

My words may vary, based on what transpires up to this point in the session. In order to provide you with some guidelines, I again offer a few alternative sample scripts:

Thank you for listening. [Conflicting part] **has agreed to listen to you now. Please respond.**

[Conflicting part] **said that ...** [Summarize the conflicting part's comments]. **That part of you appreciates that you were willing to listen, and is now willing to listen to you in return. What do you have to say in response?**

How do you respond to what you just heard?

What do you wish to say to [conflicting part]**?**

Thank you for listening. [Conflicting part] **has agreed to listen to you now. How do you feel about the job that part is doing?**

Depending on the response, I may or may not ask any additional questions regarding the motivating part's primary purpose. Use your best discretion to determine when you have sufficient information, or to continue to obtain additional insight through further discussion with the motivating part. While additional information can sometimes be helpful, I often thank this part for communicating and move on to Step 7 by asking the conflicting part to respond.

7.1.2 Calling out the conflicting part

When the motivating part emerges first, my format varies from the other scenario. In addition to repeating Steps 1 through 4, it is usually necessary to proceed through Step 5 just as though the conflicting part emerged first before asking it to respond to the motivating part (as described in Chapter 6). When I obtain sufficient information, my questions are the same as for the motivating part. After repeating the first five steps, use the same scripts provided above.

7.1.3 Calling out a third part

My first advice regarding calling out additional parts is to avoid it unless necessary. After both the conflicting and motivating parts express themselves to their satisfaction, move right on to Step 7.

In the summer of 2002, while facilitating a workshop in Ireland, the participants broke up into small groups for supervised practice late Saturday afternoon. As I approached one small group, a frustrated therapist was getting nowhere fast with five vocal parts in his client. When he first arrived at Step 6, he extended to all willing parts the opportunity to emerge, and this resulted in a parts party! His client's personality parts enjoyed themselves at the expense of his time and comfort during this breakaway practice session.

He finally asked the various parts to agree to continue the next day, and integrated them one by one. On Sunday, a female therapist helped the volunteer from the day before to resolve her initial concern by allowing only the relevant parts to speak. The client had a background in psychology, and she complimented the other therapist for the way she handled the session.

I know one hypnosis instructor who believes that we should *never* call out a third part, but there are exceptions that may benefit some of the clients some of the time. Occasionally the conflicting and motivating parts cannot attain inner resolution without the assistance of a third part, which will be explained later in this chapter.

When an exception causes me to intentionally call out a third part, this normally happens during one of the later steps. I repeat the first five steps if necessary, limiting Step 5 to asking the part's name (or title) and discovering its primary purpose. Next, I usually ask how that part can help the other parts resolve their differences, and listen to the response while taking notes. Further discussion of this appears in the last section of this chapter, and where appropriate in later chapters.

Occasionally, a third part may reveal itself spontaneously, without being called out. I deal with what emerges and immediately ask its name or title. Next I wish to know its primary purpose and why that part wants to speak. My question contains words such as, "What job do you do for John, and how can you help Happy and Success resolve their differences?"

7.1.4 Calling out a part repeatedly

During the remaining steps of parts therapy, we may repeatedly go back and forth between (or among) the parts that participate in the therapeutic process. As mentioned earlier, knowing the names (or titles) of each participating part makes this process much easier for both therapist and client. I simply address the part, calling it by name (or title) as if it were a person. Once we call out a part that has previously spoken, we are ready for the next step.

7.2 Step 7: Mediate and negotiate

Now the fun begins! Mediation and negotiation will often result in a few surprises.

This step may sometimes try your patience to the outer limits and prove your ability to deal with what emerges. Many clients have discordant parts that need to complain first to a third party, and then to each other. Often a part will talk *directly to me* rather than to the other part, even though it knows the other part is listening.

Although I endeavor to *mediate* throughout the *entire* parts therapy process, I put special emphasis on the word *mediate* here in Step 7. Proper facilitation of this step results in the client's feeling empowered, because the resolution will emerge from the client's own mind rather than from me.

7.2.1 Listen and mediate

After calling out the second part and soliciting its response to the first emerging part, I again call out the first part and ask it to respond to the second one. My initial question to John, our sample client, is short and simple: "Happy, how do you respond to Success?"

Before we start asking questions that help negotiate terms of agreement, we must first allow the parts in conflict to sufficiently vent when appropriate, and endeavor to facilitate mutual understanding between (or among) the participating parts. We may need to go back and forth several times until the motivating and conflicting parts show some willingness to understand each other's position.

I can provide no additional scripts for this portion of the mediation beyond the first question, because my questions or comments at the start of Step 7 are based on whatever each part expresses. Listening is a prerequisite to understanding; and each part must feel that the therapist and the other parts are truly listening. In other words, *each part must have the opportunity to speak and be heard.*

Be prepared for a lively dialogue! Parts often criticize either the client or other parts. While you might sometimes agree with the criticism, I cannot overemphasize the importance of remaining objective. If any participating part feels that the therapist is taking sides, the remainder of the therapeutic process becomes more difficult. Worse, if we criticize a part, we can kiss rapport goodbye; and the criticized part may become uncooperative. One of my former students found this out the hard way when a client suddenly emerged from hypnosis and resisted all subsequent induction attempts until an apology was given.

Clients may show a variety of emotions during this phase of therapy (as well as the entire therapeutic process), laughing at themselves, swearing at themselves, and/or expressing surprise at what they say about themselves. I once facilitated parts therapy in my classroom with a professional woman who used "trucker's language" during the session! Her classmates were quite surprised at the four-letter words spoken loudly before both the motivating and conflicting parts reached terms of agreement.

The length of time varies from client to client before I start negotiating. When possible, I move into this phase immediately after calling out the second part and verifying its purpose. This respects the value of my client's time and pocketbook.

7.2.2 How to negotiate

No clear line exists between mediation and negotiation, because of frequent overlap with the fifth step. Often the parts begin negotiating on their own when responding to questions about their purpose. When the parts spontaneously reveal what they wish each other to do, this makes our job much easier; but, when this information remains hidden, we must bring it forward. When appropriate, I begin the negotiations with questions. The first part I negotiate with may be either the motivating part or the conflicting part, depending on previous discussion.

We may need to go back and forth several times between the two parts, asking one or more questions of each part in conflict. Let's continue with our sample session with John right where we left off earlier in this chapter, when Success said: "... and I know that John would be happier if he could get rid of thirty pounds."

Therapist: Then what would you like Happy to do?

Success: Back off on the eating already! Enough is enough, and it is more than enough when John carries around the weight of a sack of potatoes every day. I want Happy to back off on the snacks, and to give John pleasure in achieving his goals, and in eating the right amounts of food.

Therapist: Thank you for responding. Will you now please listen while Happy speaks again?

Success: Of course.

Therapist: Happy, did you hear what Success said?

Happy: Yes.

Therapist: How do you respond to Success?

Happy: As I said before, all John wants to do is work, work, work, and there is more to life than just work. He claims to be happy with his work, yet he never takes time for himself. He always finds time to help an employee, or his wife, or his church. But, unless he starts taking some personal time for personal pleasure, I'll give him pleasure in the only way he will let me: snacks. He is only partly happy, but he hardly ever takes time to have fun.

Therapist: What would it take for you to honor Success's request? What would you like Success or John to do for you?

Happy: I want him to take one Saturday per month to play golf, or if the weather is bad he can play cards with the boys. And I want two evenings weekly for fantasy role-play games on the computer. He totally enjoys this, but feels guilty whenever he indulges—and, if he doesn't play once in a while, I'll tantalize his taste buds even more, until he gets so big that he has to buy a new wardrobe.

Therapist: Thank you for expressing. Success, how do you respond to Happy?

Success: Well, I suppose we can fit one Saturday a month into the schedule if it's that important to John's happiness, but I don't know about setting aside two evenings per week for computer games.

Therapist: Happy, how do you feel about that?

Happy: I'll compromise with one night per week average, but if he skips one week then he must give himself two nights the following week to make up for it.

Therapist: That sounds fair to me. Success, is that fair?

Success: Yeah, I guess it is.

Here are some additional examples ...

[Other part] **said that** ... [Summarize other part's purpose and complaints]. **What would you like** [other part] **to do?**

If [other part] **does what you want, what are you willing to do in return?**

What are you willing to do for [other part] **in exchange for your wishes?**

Make note of the response. Ask that part to listen while you address the other part, and choose an appropriate question similar to the following examples.

[First part] **said that** ... [Summarize first part's purpose and requests]. **How do you respond?**

What would you like [first part] **to do?**

[First part] **said that he/she is willing to** ... [Summarize what that part offered to do]. **What are you willing to do in return?**

If [first part] **does what you want, what are you willing to do in return?**

[First part] **wants you to** ... [Summarize what first part wants]. **What would you like** [first part] **to do in return?**

When we receive satisfactory responses to the above questions, we may have already completed Step 8 (*Ask parts to come to terms of agreement*) for that part. Often one or both of the conflicting parts spontaneously reach terms of agreement during Step 7, but detours often emerge. Let's discuss them before moving on.

7.3 Possible detours

While progressing on what appears to be the road to resolution, we often encounter more unexpected detours. Let's explore the common ones now, and how I get past them. This chapter section could easily be called: "Deal with what emerges".

7.3.1 The wrong part emerges

Occasionally we may attempt to call out the motivating part (or the conflicting part) and discover that another part emerges instead. There is usually a reason why another part wants to speak and be involved in the parts therapy process, so I go through Step 5 just as if talking with the first part that emerged. The additional part might be one that helps either the motivating part or the conflicting part; or its job may be neutral, yet it can often provide assistance in helping the other parts arrive at terms of agreement.

7.3.2 Dealing with mistrust

It is quite common for some parts not to trust other parts in conflict with them, and/or to hotly criticize another part. Maintaining the role of a *mediator* becomes very important here, as we must remain nonjudgmental even when a part says something that seems ridiculous. Once it is discovered, we should address mistrust promptly.

The most common mistrust takes place between the motivating and conflicting parts. Let's assume that Success says, "I don't trust Happy." In such a case the detour becomes obvious. Although it's common for one part to openly state that it does not trust another part, mistrust more often presents itself indirectly. Caustic criticism normally indicates lack of trust, and we should objectively deal with what emerges.

In the early 1990s, I saw a devout Christian who apparently never swore, but her conflicting part used vulgar language filled with four-letter words to describe its opinion of the motivating part. It had no trust whatsoever for the part that encouraged her to change. The motivating part shared the same mistrust. Before negotiating terms of agreement, it was necessary to discover when and why those two parts started mistrusting each other. This resulted in a spontaneous regression. Afterwards, when one part reached out to compromise, the other part accepted and made a counteroffer.

An inexperienced therapist might be tempted to side in with what seems like justifiable criticism and give posthypnotic suggestions too soon, but the parts could resist the suggestions and break rapport. Listen carefully when the complaining starts, and ask questions appropriately. The cause(s) often must be discovered before proceeding further. At least some degree of trust must be established before we can successfully negotiate terms of agreement between the parts in conflict.

On occasion, I can avoid discovering the original cause of the mistrust with a question such as:

"What will it take for you to trust [other part]**?"**

If that fails to provide satisfactory results, then we should continue with the other "W" questions to discover when and why the parts began mistrusting each other:

"Why don't you trust [other part]**?"**

"When did this mistrust start [etc., etc.]**?"**

"Is it possible for you to trust [other part] **a little bit?"** (This appropriate leading question is designed to elicit a yes reply. Regardless of the response, ask …)

"What can [other part] **do to earn some of your trust?"**

Note the similarity between the last question in this list and the one offered above the list: "What will it take for you to trust [other part]?" Both are designed to enable you to get back on the path leading towards negotiations and leave the detour behind. Once the parts indicate an effort to openly communicate with each other, even through stating what the other part(s) must do to earn back any broken trust, this becomes a part of future terms of agreement.

Although I can often attain sufficient resolution of mistrust without calling out additional parts, amicable negotiations sometimes seem light years away. In such circumstances, I ask:

Is there another part that you trust who is willing to speak? If so, please say "Yes" or move the yes finger. *(See next chapter section for guidance from here.)*

Sometimes, the lack of trust does not become apparent until the parts refuse to negotiate. Also, there are times when the parts do trust each other to do their respective jobs, but one (or both) might be unwilling to compromise or cooperate with the other.

7.3.3 When parts refuse to negotiate

When two parts in conflict refuse to negotiate, I normally break the deadlock by calling out a third part.

Let's assume that John's parts continue pointing the finger at each other and refuse to respond to any negotiations. First, I ask Happy and Success to agree to remain silent and listen while I invite another part to come forward and speak. Then, I continue by saying the following:

Happy and Success cannot seem to find a way to resolve their differences. Is there another part of John that can offer some suggestions or assistance? If so, please say yes or move the yes finger.

Here are more sample questions for your consideration in such circumstances.

Is there another part of [client name] **that can offer some suggestions? If so, please let me know by saying "I am here" or by moving the yes finger.**

Is there another part of [client name] **that can assist** [part name]**? If so, please say yes or indicate your presence by moving the yes finger.**

I would like to ask that part of [client name] that can offer helpful suggestions to come forward and join in the discussion. The other parts will listen. When you are ready to speak, please say "I am here" or move the yes finger.

I would like to call out that part of [client name] that has the best inner wisdom to come forward and speak. The other parts will listen.

There is a part of [client name] that can share suggestions for the other parts to consider, and they have agreed to listen. When you are ready to speak, please say "I am here" or move the yes finger.

When a part emerges, go quickly through Steps 3 and 4:

Thank you for participating. What name or title do you wish for me to call you by?

If the part gives me a proper name, I usually ask about its purpose. Frequently it gives me a title that provides a clue to its purpose, making it possible to return immediately to Step 7 with a question similar to the ones below:

How can we resolve these differences?

What suggestions do you have for the other parts?

How can you help the other parts to come to terms of agreement?

What words of wisdom do you have to offer?

What do you suggest each part do for the other?

How can the other parts find agreement?

What can each part do for the other?

What should each part expect from each other?

Listen to the answers provided by the third part, and then ask both the motivating and conflicting parts for their responses to the third part. Frequently this will get the client past the detour and back on the road to resolution.

7.3.4 *Negative or uncooperative parts*

Occasionally, a negative (or disowned) part will claim a negative job function, such as creating guilt, and refuse to cooperate or nego-tiate. After exploring the cause(s) of that part's negative purpose, I ask if it is willing to take on a new job for the client (see the next chapter for sample scripts). If so, then suggestions for a new job can come either from that part or from another part that has already been called out. Once that part agrees to a new job, I ask if it wishes a new name. Frequently, the new name generates as much enthusi-asm as the opportunity to accept a new primary purpose for the client. A previously disowned part that changes its job is usually glad to become accepted by the other parts. Although the process can sometimes be long, the results are usually worth the extra patience and effort.

On rare occasions, a part refuses to cooperate with the therapist. We must keep the ego in check and avoid arguing, which may result in a no-win situation. If a part is totally uncooperative, we may call out whatever part has the highest wisdom and ask its assistance. After thanking the part for emerging, I ask for words of wisdom or advice to help resolve the conflict. Experience demonstrates that a surprising amount of wisdom may emerge from the client, which often helps the parts in conflict come to terms of agreement. Usually, the suggestions given by this wiser part make it easy to complete Step 8.

Rather than seek innovative ways to help the parts resolve their inner conflicts, some therapists assume that a negative part is an entity and attempt to dismiss it or cast it out. Assuming that a dis-owned part is an entity is, in my opinion, inappropriate leading. Unfortunately, some therapists ask leading questions such as, "Are you a possessing or influencing entity?" In my professional opin-ion, this type of question is just as likely to cause confabulation as asking a client in hypnotic regression if her father touched her in a sexual way.

Several of my students once witnessed a psychotherapist trying to keep an ego states therapy session from falling apart after he argued with an uncooperative part. When the negative part swore at him, he assumed that it was an entity and tried to destroy it. The session ended a few minutes later with the client's inner conflicts still unresolved. Later I learned his client had been physically abused by her father; and this part was there to protect her from abusive men who might try to force their will on her.

There is a saying as old as the Scriptures: "Seek and you shall find." If you go looking for an entity, you shall surely find one, even if only in the imagination of the therapist and the person in hypnosis. I prefer to look for constructive parts, and to seek ways to persuade a disowned part to take on a constructive job for the client. That being said, I occasionally deal with a part that actually claims to be an entity when I ask about its name, title, or purpose. Rather than discuss this unusual detour here, I'll save it for Chapter 12. Meanwhile, let's continue exploring the remaining steps.

Chapter 8
Terms of Agreement

Now that the parts have expressed their complaints and concerns about each other, it's time to help them reach and confirm mutually acceptable terms of agreement. Although the next two steps frequently blend together, Step 8 often happens spontaneously during the negotiations (as mentioned in the last chapter). The analytical therapist will find that Step 9 becomes more clearly defined, but we shall explore both of these steps in one chapter. During both of these steps, we may encounter the same detours mentioned in the last chapter. Refer to that chapter for ways around those detours, and in this chapter I'll cover a few additional ones that were not previously discussed.

8.1 Step 8: Ask parts to come to terms of agreement

The goal of this step is to help the parts reach terms of agreement. During Step 7, we should pay attention to whether terms of agreement are reached spontaneously by one or both of the parts in conflict. Careful listening helps the therapist determine when each part agrees to honor the requests of the other part(s) involved. Step 8 is not complete until each conflicting part has agreed to do something constructive for the client, and has accepted all other agreements offered by any other part that was called out.

When necessary, the therapist must guide the conflicting parts into terms of agreement. This may be accomplished either by simple request, or by asking each part to offer a compromise to the other part(s) involved. Asking the parts to come up with their own solutions is more empowering than the facilitator's suggesting specific details of what each part should agree to do, and is what I call *client-centered parts therapy*.

8.1.1 What to ask

The therapist should remember the role of a mediator: *ask the right questions*, and *stay as objective as possible while looking out for the best interests of the client*. Good notes are essential during this step unless your memory is excellent, as you may need to refer to them in the ninth step. Let's continue our sample session with John, moving from Step 7 right into the eighth step.

> **Therapist:** Then let's be specific. If Happy backs off on the evening snacks, do you agree to set aside one evening per week average for computer games, and do you also agree to spend one Saturday per month either at golf or playing cards with the boys?
>
> **Success:** Yes, I suppose that is acceptable to me.
>
> **Therapist:** Happy, if Success does that for you, then are you willing to honor his request for you to stop the evening snacks?
>
> **Happy:** There is no need for me to waste time snacking just for pleasure if John gives himself the pleasure of having personal fun more often. I can make him happy having fun!
>
> **Therapist:** Then do we have an agreement?
>
> **Happy:** Yes.
>
> **Therapist:** Success, are you satisfied with this agreement, and will you honor your part?
>
> **Success:** Yes.

In a simple session with the first seven steps completed properly, Step 8 can be completed as easily as shown above. I've witnessed this many times over the years. Here are some typical questions that may result in easily completing Step 8:

What would it take for you to honor [other part]**'s request?**

If you do what [other part] **asks, what do you want in return?**

If [other part] **does what you want, what are you willing to do in return?**

Can you make a compromise with [other part]?

[Other part] wants you to [summarize the wishes of the other part] ... How much are you willing to do if [other part] agrees to do what you ask?

Are you willing to meet [other part] in the middle?

What you say or ask next depends on the responses to one of the above questions. We cannot accomplish everything exactly according to defined questions and scripts. At times, you may need to follow your intuition. Charles Tebbetts taught that good hypnotherapy is a matter of trial and error, changing, adapting to the client, and always dealing with what emerges.

So what might we say when the parts in conflict fail to give satisfactory responses to the above questions? Remember that a conflicting part may occasionally be willing to take on a *new job*. Some of the questions we may ask are as follows:

If [other part] does what you ask, are you willing to take on a new job?

If [client name or other part] loves and accepts you, are you willing to take on a new job?

Is there another job you can do for [client name] that will make you happy?

You are a part of [client name], and you can only reach your full potential of happiness [peace, achievement, security, or other goal] if [client name] is happy and content too. Are you willing to do something that will make [client name] happier?

If you agree to do what [other part] wants, would job would you like [other part] to do?

When we receive satisfactory responses to the above questions from all parts concerned, we may move right on to Step 9. However, parts therapy does not always take place on Easy Street. We still often encounter detours even this far along on the path.

8.1.2 Possible detours

In some cases of internal conflict, we may have to go for *temporary* terms of agreement and seek a permanent resolution later. Occasionally, we may have to accept a partial resolution with agreement to continue negotiations later.

Can you make a compromise until we can continue negotiations at the next session?

Are you willing to do this on a trial basis for one month, or would a one-week trial period be easier?

What are you willing to do for one week on a trial basis until our next meeting?

If you are running out of time:

We have only a little time left, but you took an important step forward today. Are you satisfied with today's progress, and are you willing to continue negotiations next week?

I wish to thank each part for expressing your concerns today, and for listening to the concerns expressed by the other part[s]. This was an important step for [client name]. However, we are running out of time, and need to continue this important communication next week. If all parts are willing to continue this progress next time, please indicate by moving the yes finger.

Remember to integrate the parts before awakening the client. At the following session, call out the same parts and continue where you left off. I will not normally terminate a session for lack of time until reaching Step 7, even if negotiations are not complete.

Sometimes we run into a total impasse rather than a detour. The first time this happened to me was in 1984, and I did something that nobody had previously taught me: *I called out a spiritual part*. During the passing years, I since learned that others were on the same page in their applications of parts therapy or its variations, giving various names to this wise part such as *inner guide, higher self, spirit guide, guardian angel*. The next chapter subsection explains more.

8.1.3 Calling out the inner wisdom

If *(and only if!)* we know in advance that our client has Christian beliefs, we may call out "the Holy Spirit inside" as a "part" to assist if needed; or we may call out that part that is most closely connected to Higher Power. Allow me to emphasize my opinion that we should work within the *client's* spiritual (or philosophical) beliefs rather than our own! If the client believes in a "higher self" concept, we may ask to speak to the "higher self" in the same manner—or a guardian angel, a spirit guide, etc. When unsure, we can ask for the "Inner Wisdom" or that part that has access to the client's highest and best wisdom.

Gordon Emmerson PhD, describes this part as the "Inner Strength" state. In the first chapter of *Ego State Therapy* (2003, page 13), he writes:

> The "Inner Strength" state (Frederick and McNeal, 1998) has many of the attributes of ego states and is referred to in some literature as an ego state (Watkins and Watkins, 1997). It may be worked with in the same manner as ego states, although there are definite differences between inner strength and ego states.

Emmerson goes on to describe the Inner Strength as a state (or part) that speaks with a clear, caring, and strong voice. In addition, it has wisdom about the purpose of the individual. My own twenty-plus years of experience validates his conclusions. Although I could write much more here about this part, I'll save it for a later chapter.

There is a part of [client name] **with inner wisdom, and can share some important ideas to consider. For** [client name]**'s benefit, please come forward and give some suggestions to help** [client name]**'s parts come to terms of agreement. When you are ready to speak, please say the words "I am here" or move the yes finger.**

No script can be provided after the above question, as we must proceed according to the response to this question. This wiser part often gets to the source of the impasse when necessary, and/or provides some wisdom to help both therapist and the parts in conflict quickly find a way to come to terms of agreement. Regardless of the name we or the client may choose or prefer, this wise part often demonstrates amazing wisdom and insight regarding the causes of a client's problem as well as the client's life purpose.

Frequently over the years, I've witnessed the wise part quickly providing the win/win compromise for two other parts that were previously unable to come to terms of agreement. Sometimes this resolution surprises both client and therapist alike. Once the solution is offered, ask each part to respond before moving on to Step 9. Very rarely do I encounter additional resistance from the parts in conflict after the Inner Strength part (or Higher Self) has spoken.

8.2 Step 9: Confirm and summarize terms of agreement

Let's assume that we now have cooperative parts that came to terms of agreement under our guidance. At a bargaining table, it would be wise for the mediator to confirm that all parties are in agreement of the terms before adjourning the meeting. The same is true for parts therapy.

Again, consider our metaphoric conflict between Roger and Linda, two employees of Company XYZ. If Roger tells Linda what he would like her to do, and vice versa, what happens if they leave the mediation table without confirming their agreements? If Roger waits for Linda to do her part before he keeps his agreement, and/or vice versa, each could slip back into old habits. They might have to return to the bargaining table at a later date. In other words, it would be wise for the mediator to confirm the agreements with all parties concerned before adjourning the meeting.

We may also consider Step 9 to be similar to closing a sale. Through questioning and probing, the sales professional eventually discovers exactly what the customer needs, and then asks for a decision. Once the customer gives a verbal approval for a product or service, the sale is confirmed only when that customer either pays money or promises to pay by signing a written agreement. The parts therapy facilitator in a sense closes the sale with each part by summarizing both the benefits and the specifics of the agreements made, and then by asking for confirmation (the verbal contract).

Words such as the following may be helpful:

[Part name or title], **you agreed to** [summarize agreements made by the part you are addressing]. **In exchange,** [other part] **has agreed to** [summarize agreements made by the other part, and any additional potential benefits]. **Are you satisfied with the agreements reached here today?**

Wait for response.

Proceed with all participating parts in the same manner as above.

Once I believe that each part will honor its agreements, I then *confirm* the terms of agreement with all the parts (as well as the conscious mind) by asking an additional question such as:

Are *all* the parts of [client name] **satisfied with the agreements reached here today? Please indicate by moving the appropriate finger, or by speaking.**

Instead of asking each part to respond individually, you may simply make a summary statement addressing each part, and then ask for the subconscious to signal confirmation of terms of agreement, such as in my sample session with John:

> **Therapist:** Success, you have agreed to set aside one Saturday monthly for either golf or for playing cards with the boys, and you have agreed to set aside an average of one evening per week for fantasy role-play games on the computer. In exchange, Happy has agreed to back off on the evening snacks and to make John happy by enjoying the occasional computer games, golf, and cards. If all parts accept the terms of agreement, please indicate either by moving the yes finger or raising your hand.

If the answer to the last question is in the affirmative (as it was with John), I proceed to Step 10. Otherwise, I give an important invitation to all the parts before moving on.

Is there any other part that wishes to express itself?

Earlier in this book, I recommended that we avoid calling out a third part unless necessary; but in rare instances a part that has not been called out might have an objection to the agreements made by the other parts. Nonverbal clues may also indicate this possibility, such as facial expressions and/or hesitation while confirming the terms of agreement. If there is a no response to the above invitation, we may proceed directly to the next step; otherwise, we must prepare for another detour.

8.2.1 Possible detours

The affirmative response makes it easy for me to know that another part wishes to emerge. I then call it out and discover its purpose, as well as what it wishes to say. After I've thanked it for emerging, my question about its purpose is short and simple: "What job do you do?" Unless the response warrants repeating all the previous parts therapy steps, my next question is:

What do you wish to say to [client name] **or the other parts?**

When the part responds, we should listen and take more notes. No script can tell us what to say next. Sometimes, the response is positive, filled with compliments to the other parts, and we can get right back on the path to Step 10. When the response is negative, my advice is to deal with what emerges and proceed accordingly.

Occasionally, there is a total absence of response to the invitation for another part wishing to express. When this occurs, I paraphrase the question to verify confirmation of the terms of agreement, but without the option to answer verbally, such as the following example:

Do all parts of [client name] **accept the terms of agreement reached here today? Please indicate with the appropriate finger response.**

Naturally, if the client responds in the affirmative, it's time for Step 10. If the client fails to respond to the above question a second time, or moves the no finger, I attempt to call out the part that objects. Here are some sample questions, which we should use only when necessary. Come up with your own questions if you wish, using my examples only as a guide.

Is there a part of [client name] who has concerns about the agreements reached here today? If so, please feel free to come forward and express yourself. We will listen. When you are ready to speak, please say the words "I am here" or move the yes finger.

I would like to talk to that part of [client name] who has concerns about the terms of agreement. Please feel free to come forward and express yourself. We will listen. When you are ready to speak, please say the words "I am here" or move the yes finger.

If a part emerges, repeat as many steps as necessary. If no part emerges, my next move is to call out the Inner Strength part in a manner similar to that described earlier in this chapter:

There is a part of [client name] with inner wisdom, and knows whether any part is objecting to the agreements reached here today. For [client name]'s benefit, and for the benefit of the parts that have made their agreements in good faith, please come forward and enlighten us. When you are ready to speak, please say the words "I am here" or move the yes finger.

If I already know that the client believes in God or a Higher Power, I may ask the following instead:

I would like to ask that part most closely connected to God or [client name]'s Higher Power to come forward if permitted. [Client name] needs your assistance in attaining resolution here today. When you are willing to speak, please say the words "I am here" or move the yes finger.

Again, the wisdom of this part may be surprisingly profound. Once a part emerges, I thank it for emerging and ask its name or title. My investigation of its primary purpose is also limited to asking, "What job do you do?"

Unless the response warrants another detour, I get straight to the point by asking:

There is a part of [client name] that prevented him/her from confirming acceptance of the agreements reached here today. Can you tell us why?

The best advice I can give here is to *ask questions* and *listen carefully* to the responses. Depending on the information learned, you may need to repeat several previous parts therapy steps before finally moving on to the tenth one. Although detours such as the ones described here are sometimes frustrating, dealing with them when they appear may be very important to the client's long-term success. It is my opinion that we need a *clear confirmation of the terms of agreement* before giving posthypnotic suggestions to the parts.

You may occasionally encounter a detour not mentioned in this book. My best advice comes in the words of the late Charles Tebbetts: "Deal with what emerges." We should also remember where we are within the eleven-step process and move on to the next step only when appropriate.

I should also note that my late mentor confirmed the terms of agreement in a very simple metaphoric way. Charlie would simply ask the parts to shake hands on their agreements. Charles Tebbetts grew up in a generation where a handshake was a man's bond and often carried more strength that the written contract. In this generation of broken promises, I prefer to be more thorough in confirming the terms of agreement. That being said, Charlie got results doing it his way, but this was in the 1970s and 1980s. Perhaps my own experience makes me a little more conservative in my approach, but I prefer to avoid leaving back doors open that might permit a part to back out of its agreement. If you wish to try it his way, do so; then, if you encounter problems, do it my way.

Chapter 9
The Final Steps

A number of practitioners of parts therapy or its variations bring the client out of hypnosis immediately after helping the parts (or ego states) come to terms of agreement, whether or not those terms are confirmed. Psychologists and psychotherapists experienced with parts therapy or its variations might find this acceptable if they are also qualified to help their clients or patients deal with any unexpected complications. However, it is my professional opinion that anyone without extensive experience in parts therapy or its variations would be wise to continue with the final steps presented in this chapter and follow the parts therapy process with suggestions and imagery. Including these additional steps will minimize the risk of setbacks and/or interference from one or more parts, thus giving the client a greater probability of long-term resolution.

9.1 Step 10: Give direct suggestion as appropriate

Once the parts confirm their terms of agreement, we may give posthypnotic suggestions both before and after integration. While our choices broaden after the final step of parts therapy, we need to be more specific prior to integration. In other words, my suggestions given prior to integration are direct suggestions given to each participating part. Additionally, all suggestions given *before* Step 11 should relate to the terms of agreement reached, along with confidence to do so, coupled with direct suggestions for the parts to cooperate.

I paraphrase the terms of agreement by giving each part instructions to keep its promises. These specific suggestions detail the agreements made, while encouraging each part to follow through on its promises. Although some circumstances may warrant indirect suggestions, I use direct suggestions with most clients during Step 10.

My normal modus operandi is to simply address each part individually and review the specifics of the agreements previously confirmed, much as a mediator might do before concluding a successful mediation. It makes no difference whether we address the conflicting part first or the motivating part first. My choice is often intuitive, but sometimes it is based on which part shows the greater rapport. It would be almost impossible to script every suggestion to give during this step; but perhaps the following samples might help you get started.

First, I would like to thank all the parts involved for this open communication and great progress made here today.

Continue with one or more of the following ...

Also, [part name or title], **thank you for agreeing to help** [client name and/or other part] ... [repeat that part's agreement]. **Every day in every way you find it easier and easier to keep your agreement.** [Get as specific as possible; then repeat the above with each participating part.]

[Client name] **will be happier because of the agreement you made here today, and you are a part of** [client name]. **So you will also be happier by helping** [client name or part name] **to ...** [restate the terms, and be specific].

If working together with another part ...

Also, by working with [other part's name], **it becomes even easier for you to honor the agreement made here today.** [Give appropriate suggestions.]

You may give any other suggestions that are in total harmony with the terms of agreement. In rare instances it might be appropriate to use guided imagery to the parts during Step 10. Normally, I do this only if the client has created his/her guided imagery during the parts therapy process, and then said imagery remains compatible with any imagery previously supplied by the client.

Here is what I said during my sample session with John …

> **Therapist:** Happy, every day in every way you find it easier and easier to allow John to be satisfied eating the right amounts of the right food. You know that you can enjoy making him happy having fun at the computer as planned, and he has one Saturday per month to enjoy either golf or cards. You can be even happier knowing that John will enjoy living a more balanced life. Success, you will now honor your agreement with Happy, allowing John to play fantasy role-play games once weekly. He can also play golf or cards once monthly. You can feel a sense of achievement knowing that John will be happy scheduling occasional time for play, and this is just as important as planning other activities at work or home. By allowing Happy to make John happy having fun occasionally, you may find it easier to motivate John to achieve all his important goals in life.

It's time to bring this closer to home. Let's assume your client had a part that wanted to smoke (Smoky) and a part that wanted to quit (Healthy). After an initial impasse, a third part suggested that the client continue to smoke, but do so occasionally and use moderation in all things. Smoky agreed to smoke only once after each meal, and at no other times; and Healthy agreed to smoke in moderation rather than trying to abstain totally as in the past. What would you say to the parts after confirming their terms of agreement? Jot down your notes before peeking at the suggestions revealed in Chapter 11. Before writing down your ideas for the smoker above, note that I do not give posthypnotic suggestions to a part that did not make any agreements, although I still thank such a part for participating in the session.

Out of fairness to the late Charles Tebbetts, I should mention that he frequently gave direct suggestions to the parts before confirming the terms of agreement, thus reversing the order of Steps 9 and 10. Although it may not make any difference to the client, I'm more comfortable following the steps in the order presented in this book, and I teach my students to do likewise. Now let's move on the Step 11.

9.2 Step 11: Integrate the parts

While a number of practitioners of the variations of parts therapy bring the client out of hypnosis without integrating the parts (or ego states), I follow the example of Charles Tebbetts by integrating the parts into a harmonious whole. He used the metaphor of the conscious mind as resembling a symphony conductor, and the parts were members of the orchestra playing their various instruments to create harmonious music. The conscious mind makes the decisions and the parts follow the lead, just as the violinists and other musicians follow the conductor. If two musicians play out of tune or have a conflict, once they know what notes to play, they take their respective seats and blend back in with the rest of the orchestra. Although I occasionally use Charlie's metaphor while teaching parts therapy to my students, I rarely do so with my clients.

Before integration, Tebbetts would usually ask the parts to embrace or to hold hands etc. for mutual love and acceptance. Then he would ask the client to allow all the parts to merge into an integrated or complete whole, and to *confirm* when the integration was complete by raising a hand. After some posthypnotic suggestions, he concluded the session.

I've already discussed my more thorough way of confirming the terms of agreement and giving direct suggestion as appropriate. Then, when I'm ready to integrate the parts, I simply thank the parts for their cooperation (if not done previously), and give suggestions for them to integrate into a harmonious whole in a manner similar to that of my late friend and mentor. Also, I ask the client to indicate when it is done.

Here is how to integrate Happy and Success in our sample session ...

> **Therapist:** And now, I'd like to ask both Success and Happy to shake hands, and to integrate into a harmonious whole. John can remain aware of these two parts, with each part honoring the agreements made here today. And, when the parts are integrated into a harmonious whole, please indicate either by moving the yes finger or saying, "It is done."
>
> **Client:** It is done.
>
> **Therapist:** Excellent. You have done well. And now imagine that you are already at your ideal weight, doing one of your favorite activities. Imagine your benefits ... [etc.].

My words may vary slightly from client to client. Here are some additional examples of what to say:

Now it's time for all the parts to integrate into inner harmony, and when this integration is complete, please either move the yes finger or raise your hand.

I would like to thank all the parts for the excellent progress today, which will benefit [client name] greatly. Your cooperation was greatly appreciated, and [client name] will be much happier now. When you are ready to merge into a harmonious whole, please do so, and indicate when this is done either by moving the yes finger or raising your hand.

Will all parts hold hands or embrace now? Thank you. And, when you are integrated into a state of inner harmony, please indicate by moving the yes finger or by raising your hand.

We may also ask the client to imagine seeing, hearing, or simply *feeling* when this inner harmony or integration is complete. Then, we should make it easy for them to give confirmation when it is done.

When you see your parts to integrate into a harmonious whole, or when the parts tell you it is done, please move the yes finger or say, "It is done."

Please ask all your parts to integrate into a harmonious whole. When you feel [know, sense etc.] that the integration is complete, or when the parts tell you it is done, please move the yes finger or say, "It is done."

I normally wait at least thirty seconds for a response before repeating the question in different words. If there is no response the second time, then I move back and ask if there is any part that wishes to express. So far, with over twenty years of experience in parts therapy, the occasional times that a client has failed to confirm integration have *always* resulted in the emergence of another part. Based on the time frame, I will either deal with what emerges at that time, or ask the parts to agree to continue at the next session. When it is necessary to wait until a later session, I'll then ask the part that just emerged if it is willing to integrate until called out at the next meeting. Again, by treating every part with courtesy and respect as though it were a separate person, we will find that cooperation will normally be easy to obtain.

When I obtain confirmation of the integration, this concludes the parts therapy process itself; but normally I'm not quite ready to bring the client out of hypnosis until I have given some additional suggestions.

9.3 *Give additional suggestions and/or guided imagery*

For many years I taught students that additional suggestions represented the twelfth step of parts therapy, as shown in the first two editions of my book, *The Art of Hypnotherapy*. Not until 2003 did one of my students correctly point out the fact that the formal parts therapy process is complete with integration at Step 11. In other words, giving additional suggestions becomes part of the *conclusion* to the hypnotherapy session, just as the induction, deepening, establishing ideomotor responses etc. are included as part of the preparation.

If time permits, we may use an appropriate prepared script and/or guided imagery that relates to the client's goal, emphasizing his/her personal benefits. Even if time has run out, it's usually a good idea to give at least one or two therapeutic posthypnotic suggestions to reinforce subconscious relearning before awakening in order to reinforce the progress made during the parts therapy process. For smokers or clients on weight reduction, I often reinforce their personal benefits with guided imagery and indirect suggestions before awakening the client. Suggestions (both direct and indirect) are customized to each particular client.

Now let's review some important information. Remember the four hypnotherapy objectives from Chapter 3? They are: *suggestion and imagery, discovering the cause, release,* and *subconscious relearning*. Competent facilitation of the eleven-step process of parts therapy should accomplish the second and third of these objectives before integration of the parts. Good positive suggestions (the first objective) may then enhance subconscious relearning (the fourth objective) after the formal parts therapy process is complete. Thus, a complete hypnosis session including client-centered parts therapy accomplishes all four of the hypnotherapy objectives.

9.4 Concluding the session

When appropriate, I awaken the client. Students familiar with my training program know that I use a very slow awakening procedure, especially when a client has experienced a deep level of trance. A rapid wake-up procedure could leave some clients with a headache, especially if they are emerging from deeper states. (I know this from personal experience after being awakened abruptly once.) My awakening normally takes 45 to 60 seconds while I count slowly from one to five:

Now, I'm going to start counting from one up to five, bringing you back to full conscious awareness.

Number one ... Beginning to emerge from hypnosis now, starting your journey back from hypnosis into full conscious awareness. Every nerve and muscle feels good, as though you have taken a very pleasant, relaxing hypnotic nap ... and you feel wonderfully good.

Number two ... Slowly, calmly, gently and gradually, you are becoming more and more aware of this room, the chair you are sitting on, and where you are.

Number three ... Whenever you get behind the wheel of a motor vehicle, you are totally alert in every way, responding appropriately to any and all traffic and road situations.

Number four ... Beginning to stretch your muscles if you wish, allowing a wonderful, rejuvenating energy to flow from head to toe.

Number five, open your eyes. Take a deep breath, and feel good in every way!

Remember that clients normally remain in rapport with the hypnotist for several minutes after emerging from hypnosis, and may be very open to suggestions. For this reason, we need to choose our words wisely. My first words are something like, "Did you surprise yourself?" or "Are you happy with your resolution?" After the response, I keep the discussion somewhat brief unless it is the final session with that client.

In many cases, I ask the client to see me at least once more to be sure the resolution will be permanent. When backsliding indicates the need to do so, I might call out the parts again to find out which part isn't keeping the terms of agreement, and why. This is rare, but sometimes necessary. Normally at a follow-up session, the parts are honoring their agreements, so I simply reinforce the client's original goal with suggestions and imagery.

For example, I might tell a smoker, "Each day is easier than the day before, and each week easier than the week before ... until it becomes so easy that you feel as though you've always been a non-smoker ... and it simply becomes easier than you thought possible. Every time you take a deep breath at times you used to light up, you reinforce your power of choice. Each time you make a wise choice, it becomes easier to make another wise choice, because all your parts are cooperating in *inner harmony*. And, as a muscle that's used becomes stronger with use, your power of choice becomes stronger with use, until you have a greater strength of will than you thought possible." Clients overcoming other undesired habits receive similar empowering suggestions. For additional reinforcement at home, I may give the client either a generic or personalized hypnosis tape with various suggestions and guided imagery (unless that has been done after a previous session).

In the next chapter, we will review our entire sample session with John, and outline the typical parts therapy session.

Chapter 10
The Typical Session

Now that we have thoroughly explored the parts therapy process, let's review the entire sample session with John, and then outline a typical parts therapy session.

10.1 John: Weight reduction

This section contains the complete parts therapy process of the sample session with John (fictitious name), shown in pieces in previous chapters. Numerous clients over the years could easily identify with the sample session in this book, making it impossible to identify which client was John (or whether John was a man or woman).

In the original intake session, I explain to all clients seeing me for weight control that diets work on the body, but not on the mind. This is evident by the number of people who find their weight going up and down like a yo-yo. Unless or until the subconscious accepts a change of eating habits, the person who goes on a diet will eventually find the weight that is lost! John already experienced a session with suggestion and imagery of his personal benefits; but his subconscious rejected the positive approach, and he felt that a part of him was undermining the beneficial suggestions.

Many parts therapy sessions are simple, with a simple solution. As indicated above, the cause of John's inner conflict is a common theme I've seen numerous times over the years. We join our session with John at the beginning of the eleven-step process, after proper preparation, with the client at sufficient hypnotic depth. Without looking in earlier chapters, can you determine when I move from one step into another?

Therapist: There is a part of you that makes you snack frequently after dinner, and it is doing a very good job. I'm talking to that part of

119

John that causes him to snack frequently. You are an important part of John. There is probably a good reason for what you're doing … and you are doing a good job. John is willing to listen, and I am willing to listen. I'm sure that you are doing what you think is right, but another part of John is unhappy, and feels that better communication can enlighten both of you with a few ideas that could make John much happier. If you would like to gain more information and communicate, John is willing to listen to whatever you have to say. When you are willing to communicate, please let us know by saying the words "I am here" or by moving the yes finger.

Conflicting part: I am here.

Therapist: Thank you for communicating.

Conflicting part: [no response.]

Therapist: What name or title do you wish to be called?

Conflicting part: I'm Happy.

Therapist: Hi, Happy! What job do you do for John?

Happy: I make him do things that make him happy.

Therapist: I see. How do you make John happy?

Happy: Well, I make him snack at night because he likes the taste of food.

Therapist: Is there anything else you do to make him happy?

Happy: No. He gets pleasure when I tantalize his taste buds.

Therapist: Why do you feel that tantalizing his taste buds is necessary in order to keep him happy?

Happy: Well, he never takes time to do anything else that makes him happy, and he deserves some happiness in life. He only seems to have time for the three "Ws".

Therapist: What are the three "Ws"?

Happy: Work, work, work!

Therapist: Would you please explain further?

Happy: Well, John is proud of his success—but he works too hard. He is so busy being a good worker, a good father, a good husband, and a good Christian that he never takes time to *enjoy* his success. What good is working to be successful if you can't take time to enjoy some of it yourself?

Therapist: Thank you for communicating. You provided some very important information. Would you be willing to listen now while I call out another part of John?

Happy: Yes.

Therapist: Thank you … and now, I'd like to talk to that part of John that motivates him to reach his ideal weight and control his eating habits. You are an important part of John, and there is probably a good reason for what you're doing … and you motivated him to invest his time and money to participate in these sessions, so you are doing a good job. Happy is willing to listen, and I'm willing to listen. When you are ready to speak, please say the words "I am here" or move the yes finger.

Motivating part: I am here.

Therapist: Thank you for communicating. What name or title should I call you?

Motivating part: I'm Success.

Therapist: Hi, Success! What job do you do for John?

Success: I motivate him to be all he can be.

Therapist: [pause … I'm listening in case Success continues.]

Success: John sets good goals, and I help him to achieve them. He is a good person, and I motivate him to stay that way.

Therapist: That's a very important job, but did you hear what Happy said?

Success: Yes.

Therapist: Thank you for listening to Happy. Happy has agreed to listen to you now, so how do you respond to what Happy said?

Success: John gets great satisfaction at being successful in business, and in having a good marriage and stable family. He always accomplishes whatever he puts his mind to do, because I'm always here to help him; but we can't seem to get that extra weight to go away because of Happy. Yet Happy says his job is to make John happy, and I know that John would be happier if he could get rid of thirty pounds.

Therapist: Then what would you like Happy to do?

Success: Back off on the eating already! Enough is enough, and it is more than enough when John carries around the weight of a sack of potatoes every day. I want Happy to back off on the snacks, and to give John pleasure in achieving his goals, and in eating the right amounts of food.

Therapist: Thank you for responding. Will you now please listen while Happy speaks again?

Success: Of course.

Therapist: Happy, did you hear what Success said?

Happy: Yes.

Therapist: How do you respond to Success?

Happy: As I said before, all John wants to do is work, work, work, and there is more to life than just work. He claims to be happy with his work, yet he never takes time for himself. He always finds time to help an employee, or his wife, or his church. But, unless he starts taking some personal time for personal pleasure, I'll give him pleasure in the only way he will let me: snacks. He is only partly happy, but he hardly ever takes time to have fun.

Therapist: What would it take for you to honor Success's request? What would you like Success or John to do for you?

Happy: I want him to take one Saturday per month to play golf, or if the weather is bad he can play cards with the boys. And I want two evenings weekly for fantasy role-play games on the computer. He totally enjoys this, but feels guilty whenever he indulges—and, if he doesn't play once in a while, I'll tantalize his taste buds even more, until he gets so big that he has to buy a new wardrobe.

Therapist: Thank you for expressing. Success, how do you respond to Happy?

Success: Well, I suppose we can fit one Saturday a month into the schedule if it's that important to John's happiness, but I don't know about setting aside two evenings per week for computer games.

Therapist: Happy, how do you feel about that?

Happy: I'll compromise with one night per week average, but if he skips one week then he must give himself two nights the following week to make up for it.

Therapist: That sounds fair to me. Success, is that fair?

Success: Yeah, I guess it is.

Therapist: Then let's be specific. If Happy backs off on the evening snacks, do you agree to set aside one evening per week average for computer games, and do you also agree to spend one Saturday per month either at golf or playing cards with the boys?

Success: Yes, I suppose that is acceptable to me.

Therapist: Happy, if Success does that for you, then are you willing to honor his request for you to stop the evening snacks?

Happy: There is no need for me to waste time snacking just for pleasure if John gives himself the pleasure of having personal fun more often. I can make him happy having fun!

Therapist: Then do we have an agreement?

Happy: Yes.

Therapist: Success, are you satisfied with this agreement, and will you honor your part?

Success: Yes.

Therapist: Success, you have agreed to set aside one Saturday monthly for either golf or for playing cards with the boys, and you have agreed to set aside an average of one evening per week for fantasy role-play games on the computer. In exchange, Happy has agreed to back off on the evening snacks and to make John happy by enjoying the occasional computer games, golf and cards. If all parts accept the terms of agreement, please indicate either by moving the yes finger or raising your hand.

[Right hand rises.]

Therapist: Is there any other part that wishes to express at this time?

[The no finger moves.]

Therapist: Happy, every day in every way you find it easier and easier to allow John to be satisfied eating the right amounts of the right food. You know that you can enjoy making him happy having fun at the computer as planned, and he has one Saturday per month to enjoy either golf or cards. You can be even happier knowing that John will enjoy living a more balanced life. Success, you will now honor your agreement with Happy, allowing John to play fantasy role-play games once weekly. He can also play golf or cards once monthly. You can feel a sense of achievement knowing that John will be happy scheduling occasional time for play, and this is just as important as planning other activities at work or home. By allowing Happy to make John happy having fun occasionally, you may find it easier to motivate John to achieve all his important goals in life.

[Pause ...]

Therapist: And now, I'd like to ask both Success and Happy to shake hands, and to integrate into a harmonious whole. John can remain aware of these two parts, with each part honoring the agreements made here today. And, when the parts are integrated into a harmonious whole, please indicate either by moving the yes finger or saying, "It is done."

Client: It is done.

Therapist: Excellent. You have done well. And now imagine that you are already at your ideal weight, doing one of your favorite activities. Imagine your benefits ... [etc.].

In retrospect, the cause of John's problem was a combination of inner conflict and present unresolved issue. He was a workaholic whose life was out of balance. (This is a common problem in the USA, where increasing professional and personal demands on our time make it difficult to live a balanced life.) This cause had to be discovered and released, along with a solution that was acceptable to both the motivating part and the conflicting part (subconscious relearning).

After the eleven-step process, additional suggestions and imagery (once called the twelfth step) enhance the relearning process. Now that we have reviewed our sample session with John, let's outline the entire process and put this former twelfth step in its proper place.

10.2 Outline of parts therapy session

If you are using this book as a text, your instructor may ask you to memorize the following outline:

A. Preparation
1. Give preinduction discussion, including explanation of parts therapy to client.
2. Choose and use appropriate hypnotic induction for client.
3. Deepen to at least medium depth, using hypnotic convincers if necessary.
4. Establish (or reconfirm) peaceful place.
5. Establish (or confirm) ideomotor-response signals (A4 and A5 may be reversed if desired).
6. Verify hypnotic depth. (I use the 100 to 1 scale with finger response).

B. Parts therapy (eleven-step process)
1. Identify the part.
2. Gain rapport (compliment the part).
3. Call out the part.
4. Thank it for emerging.
5. Discover its purpose.
6. Call out other parts as appropriate.
7. Negotiate and mediate.
8. Ask parts to come to terms of agreement.
9. Confirm and summarize terms of agreement.
10. Give direct suggestions as appropriate.
11. Integrate the parts! (The formal parts therapy process is completed.)

C. Conclusion
1. Give additional suggestions and/or guided imagery.
2. Awaken.
3. Briefly discuss therapy with client and set next appointment if appropriate.

Now that we have reviewed a sample session, as well as the outline of a typical parts therapy session, let's explore some case histories. Afterwards, we will look at some potential pits. Last but not least, we'll then boldly go where few have gone before: into the Undiscovered Country.

Chapter 11
Sample Sessions

Students and therapists alike are interested in knowing how parts therapy has successfully helped others to resolve inner conflicts.

When Charles Tebbetts wrote *Miracles on Demand*, his detailed discussion of case histories was one of the book's strongest selling points. The words spoken during sessions were preserved almost verbatim in printed form in his book. Some of his case summaries appear in a chapter in my book, *The Art of Hypnotherapy*, as well as mine, and some facilitated by my students. One of Charlie's best sessions was detailed in an entire chapter of my text, with that client's written permission.

Today, in the absence of written permission from clients, I am far more cautious regarding any details of sessions that could reveal a client's identity. (Laws are stricter now in the USA than they were before the dawn of the new millennium.) In order to illustrate effective parts therapy, I have interwoven composites of actual conversations heard during sessions, both in my earlier example of John and in the sample session of the smoker in this chapter. Most of the statements made by parts are phrases that I've heard numerous times from clients over the years. Names are also fictitious to further maintain anonymity. The case summaries that appear in my book are taken either from my demonstrations at workshops, or with students in my classes over the years, although I changed their names and occupations (except where otherwise noted). Most part names are accurate.

11.1 The smoker

Now let's explore a sample parts therapy session for a smoker trying to quit. This sample session has a few surprises and detours, based on a composite of several similar cases over the years. Again, a number of my former clients and students could easily relate to what appears below, thus preserving anonymity. We shall call our smoker Donna.

> **Therapist:** There is a part of you that makes you smoke frequently, and it is doing a very good job. I'm talking to that part of Donna that causes her to smoke. You are an important part of Donna, and there is probably a good reason for what you're doing ... and you are doing a good job. Donna is willing to listen, and I am willing to listen. I'm sure that you are doing what you think is right, but another part of Donna is unhappy, and feels that better communication can enlighten both of you. If you would like to gain more information and communicate, Donna is willing to listen to whatever you have to say. When you are willing to communicate, please let us know by saying the words "I am here" or by moving the yes finger.
>
> **Conflicting part:** I am here.
>
> **Therapist:** Thank you for communicating.
>
> **Conflicting part:** You're welcome, I think.
>
> **Therapist:** What name or title do you wish to be called?
>
> **Conflicting part:** I'm Smokey.
>
> **Therapist:** Hi, Smokey! What job do you do for Donna?
>
> **Smokey:** Well, I make sure she keeps on smoking.
>
> **Therapist:** Why do you do that?
>
> **Smokey:** Because Donna doesn't have to do what others tell her to do. She values her freedom of choice, and too many meddlers out there are trying to force her to quit.
>
> **Therapist:** I see ... so when did you first take on this job?
>
> **Smokey:** The first time her father told her to quit smoking ... he was a smoker, and he was a hypocrite for telling her not to smoke. And many of those idiots trying to ban smoking in public are ex-smokers, so what gives them the right to try to force others to quit? Every time Donna lights up, she is making a statement that she has freedom of choice.

Therapist: Is there any other job you do for her?

Smokey: Not really. This one keeps me quite busy.

Therapist: That's easy to believe, because you are doing a good job. How do you make sure she keeps on smoking?

Smokey: I do this the obvious way, by making sure she always has cigarettes handy, and making sure she responds to smoking triggers.

Therapist: Thank you for communicating. Are you willing to listen while I talk to another part of Donna?

Smokey: Yes.

Therapist: Thank you. Donna, there is another part of you that wishes to quit smoking, and she is an important part of you. I'm speaking to that part now. There is probably a good reason for what you're doing … and you motivated her to invest time and money in several stop-smoking programs, including this one. You are doing a good job. Smokey is willing to listen, and I'm willing to listen. When you are ready to speak, please say the words "I am here" or move the yes finger.

Motivating part: I am here.

Therapist: Thank you … what name or title should I call you?

Motivating part: Call me Healthy.

Therapist: Hello, Healthy, what job do you do for Donna?

Healthy: Isn't that obvious from my name? I help her stay healthy.

Therapist: How do you do that?

Healthy: Well, I motivate her to learn all she can learn about how to stay healthy. She eats well, and exercises regularly, but keeps on polluting her system with smoke.

Therapist: Did you hear what Smokey had to say?

Healthy: Of course I did, but Smokey is full of it.

Therapist: What would you like Smokey to do for you? And, if Smokey agrees, what are you willing to do for Smokey?

Healthy: Smokey needs to just get over this smoking nonsense, or get lost.

Therapist: Is there anything else you wish to say to Smokey at this time?

Healthy: No, because I doubt if Smokey would listen.

Therapist: Would you like to ask Smokey to take on a new job?

Healthy: No, because it would be fruitless. Smokey is stubborn.

Therapist: Would you listen again while I talk to Smokey?

Healthy: Yes, but I doubt that it will do any good.

Therapist: Smokey, how do you respond to Healthy?

Smokey: I don't trust Healthy, and I don't like her.

Therapist: What would it take for Healthy to earn your trust?

Smokey: She needs to back off on this nonsmoking nonsense, and that won't happen. Nobody has the right to tell Donna not to smoke. If Donna had faith the size of a grain of a mustard seed, she could smoke without getting sick—but *no*, she has to buy into the bias of people who feel they have a right to tell us how to live our lives. Healthy needs to grow up and quit telling Donna what to do.

Therapist: How can we resolve the conflict between you and Healthy?

Smokey: There is *no* way that I will quit smoking, so the question is irrelevant. If Healthy keeps on pushing me, I'll make Donna smoke three packs a day.

Therapist: Would you at least hear what Healthy has to say in response?

Smokey: Yes, but I doubt that it will do any good.

Therapist: Healthy, how do you respond to Smokey?

Healthy: Smokey is a rebellious idiot. Tell her to get lost before she destroys Donna's good health. Smokey does not belong here.

Therapist: Is there another part that can offer a solution, or give some words of wisdom? If so, please come forward and indicate your willingness by either moving the "yes" finger or saying, "I am here."

Third part: I am here.

Therapist: Thank you for emerging. What name or title should I call you?

Third part: Call me Serena.

Therapist: Hi, Serena. What job do you do for Donna?

Serena: I am Donna's Guardian Angel.

Therapist: Thank you again for being here. Have you heard what both Smokey and Healthy have said today?

Serena: Yes.

Therapist: What words of wisdom do you have to offer to help us find resolution?

Serena: Well, the impasse is because neither part has accepted the possibility of compromise. Donna can smoke five or six cigarettes daily, smoking only when she is consciously aware of each and every time she lights up. Smoking occasionally, in moderation, will be far less risky to her health than smoking heavily.

Therapist: Thank you. Healthy, how do you respond to Serena?

Healthy: I didn't think it was possible to smoke occasionally. Others have told Donna that you either do not smoke, or you are out of control. Is it really possible to smoke only a few cigarettes daily?

Therapist: Serena says that it is possible. Can you allow this?

Healthy: Yes, as long as Donna doesn't go out of control.

Therapist: Is there anything you would like to say to Serena?

Healthy: No … I trust Serena.

Therapist: Thank you. Smokey, how do you respond to Serena?

Smokey: Hallelujah! It's about time Donna listened to common sense! This is what I wanted to begin with, but nobody would listen to me—not even Donna.

Therapist: Then are you willing to allow Donna to smoke only when she consciously chooses, which is only about five or six cigarettes per day?

Smokey: Yes, gladly, as long as Healthy doesn't try to make her quit.

Therapist: Do you wish to take on a new name or new job?

Smokey: Not yet, but I'll do what Serena suggested if Healthy cooperates.

Therapist: And you will let Donna forget her urges at other times?

Smokey: Yes.

Therapist: Then we have terms of agreement from both of you? If so, move the yes finger.

[Yes finger moves.]

Therapist: You made a very important decision today! Healthy, you have agreed to permit Donna to smoke five or six times per day, only when she consciously chooses to do so. And Smokey, you have agreed to let Donna forget her urges except at the times she consciously chooses to smoke. Please confirm your acceptance of this agreement by moving the yes finger or raising your hand.

[Yes finger moves.]

Therapist: Serena, do you have anything else you wish to say?

Serena: No, except that Donna will be much happier if both parts honor their agreements. I will give both parts the strength to keep their word.

Therapist: Thank you. Is there any other part that needs to express today?

[No response.]

Therapist: Then I would like to thank all parts for their participation, and ask that Healthy and Smokey shake hands or embrace each other with mutual acceptance—and, when all parts integrate into a harmonious whole, please indicate either by moving the yes finger or by raising your hand.

[After about thirty seconds, her right hand rises.]

Therapist: Excellent. Now, whenever a situation occurs that used to trigger an automatic light-up, you may simply take ONE DEEP BREATH. Immediately, that reminds you to put your mind on whatever you choose. And you can either remember to forget the fair-weather friend, or you can forget to remember yesterday's urges ... fading into the past, forgotten in the midst of time. The key to overcoming the habitual urges is to simply enjoy your new friend FREEDOM, to think about whatever you choose! ... and you can smoke only when you consciously choose. Both Healthy and Smokey have agreed to make this reality, and, like a muscle that's used is stronger with use, your power of choice is stronger with use. Each day becomes easier than the day before, and each week becomes easier than the week before, because you LOVE your power of choice ... and with all parts working with inner harmony, you can enjoy the freedom to be the person you choose to be. And so it is.

The last paragraph above gives you an idea of how I wrap up a parts therapy session such as this. Additional suggestions may also be included, customized to the client's benefits for quitting.

Although the above is not a typical session, I've facilitated several sessions like this for smokers over the years. Occasionally, two parts in conflict will need the help of a third part before reaching terms of agreement, which often ends up being a compromise from the original goal stated by the conscious mind. Note that I endeavor to avoid the trap of letting one part persuade me to get rid of another part. (This scenario has also appeared in sessions a number of times over the years.) Rather than assume that Smokey didn't belong in Donna (as Healthy believed), I called out a third part. This is more client-centered than making assumptions that might be incorrect.

Also note that I do not take the position of forcing a smoker to quit totally if he or she decides to smoke occasionally instead. I believe that the *client is the hypnotherapist's employer*, and the therapist should endeavor to help the client's subconscious accept the changes chosen by the client. A number of smokers seeing me over the years have resolved inner conflicts by smoking in moderation rather than quitting totally. One such client told me after a similar parts therapy session that he felt less stress than at any time in over a year since making an agreement with himself to smoke occasionally instead of quitting totally. He told me he reserved the right to change his mind, and that he might choose to quit totally after a couple more years.

I need to add one final note here: in order to maintain conscious control, I recommend that the occasional smoker keep the supply of cigarettes *out of arm's reach*, so that a conscious decision must be made before getting a cigarette. At home, the supply could be kept in a kitchen drawer or bedroom drawer. In the car, the supply could be kept in the trunk, say, or glove box. This prevents automatically reaching in the shirt pocket or getting into the purse without conscious awareness.

Now let's explore two actual sessions before looking at a few session summaries. We start with another smoker.

11.2 A smoky mirror

Here is another case summary similar to the example of Donna. Jim failed repeatedly on numerous attempts to quit smoking, but had every expectation of succeeding after learning the basics of hypnosis during his certification training. Now that he understood the power of the mind, he believed that he could quit simply by having another student facilitate one or two practice sessions with his. Sometimes, however, the inner child has a way of clinging to the past.

The more he tried to quit, the greater the intensity of his inner conflict. Parts therapy revealed that he originally started smoking in order to make a statement of rebellion against a domineering parent. The conflicting part called itself Freedom, whose purpose was to make sure that Jim was free to make his own choices in life. He did that by rebelling at illogical orders, especially if given by a hypocrite. Further questions revealed that Freedom resented the hypocrisy of his mother when she said, "Do as I say, not as I do." As you might suspect, his mother was a smoker.

Freedom regressed to the first time he smoked (in his early teens). He found a pack of cigarettes on the kitchen table, and removed one. He took it into the bathroom, and gazed at his reflection in the mirror, blurred by a thin layer of moisture. After using a towel to wipe a clear spot large enough to reflect his facial image, he decided it was time to grow up. He put an unlit cigarette in his mouth and stared further at the reflection of his image, comparing it with his memory of the image of the Marlboro man.

He found a match and lit the cigarette. Although inhaling made him cough, he blew smoke at his image reflected in the mirror, making it smoky. In spite of his initial discomfort, this young teenager would prove to his mother that he was more grown up now, and by lighting up he demonstrated that he was old enough to make his own choices.

When the motivating part was called out, it took on the adult name, James. Negotiations came quickly and easily when James told Freedom that the cigarette was stealing his ability to choose the benefits of more money and good health by making him obey the urges. James reminded Freedom that he was smarter than the mindless cigarette, and that he could rebel at the urges rather than try to rebel at his late mother's orders to avoid smoking. Freedom took on the job of choosing new ways to spend the money that had previously gone up in smoke.

11.3 Unexpected cause

Debby asked me for a private session after attending a recent parts therapy workshop, and I am grateful to her for allowing me to include her session notes in this book.

Many years of obesity brought her health to a possible fork in the road. She was very intelligent and well educated. Yet, in spite of her many professional and personal accomplishments, Debby was unable to accomplish this important personal goal. Her background in both hypnotherapy and psychology resulted in a rather informative discussion before hypnosis, as she felt that the cause of her problem was rooted in two of the seven psychodynamics: past event (abandonment), and secondary gain (protection).

We initially considered the possibility of regression to deal with the feelings of abandonment, but felt that we could still use parts therapy to explore the cause(s) that were most closely related to her eating disorder. Debby also told me that, when her husband left her, she put on considerably more weight in order to protect herself from getting into another relationship.

Many hypnotherapists and psychotherapists alike could have easily used this information to take what would have been the wrong path to success.

Taking the path of client-centered parts therapy resulted in a very productive and interesting session, which I would have loved to have on videotape. The conflicting part called itself Little One. Although I gave Debby a copy of my detailed session notes, she gave me a photocopy, along with written permission to include them in this book. Let's pick up the session after I called out the conflicting part.

Conflicting part: I am here.

Therapist: Thank you for communicating. What name or title shall I call you?

Conflicting part: Little One.

Therapist: Hi, Little One. What job do you do for Debby?

Little One: I keep her content.

Therapist: How do you keep her content?

Little One: I give her the munchies. Whenever she is jealous or angry, I make her feel content.

Therapist: Why do you give her the munchies in order to make her content?

Little One: It gives her something to do, and it satisfies her. It takes her mind off of the real issues.

Therapist: Thank you. Would you be willing to listen while I call out another part?

Little One: Yes.

After identifying and calling out the motivating part …

Therapist: Thank you for emerging. What name or title shall I call you?

Motivating part: Adult.

Therapist: Hello, Adult. What is your primary purpose?

Adult: I should be in charge. I make things happen, I help Debby succeed, to stay in focus, and to achieve her desires.

Therapist: How do you do this?

Adult: When she pursues her desires, she gets things in focus, and then gets things done.

Therapist: [after confirming that Adult listened to the first part] How do you respond to Little One?

Adult: Little One gets in the way. She needs to work with me rather than against me.

Therapist: How should she do that?

Adult: She needs to stop sidetracking our effort to reduce. Debby needs to stop the excess eating! Weight should not be an issue.

Therapist: Thank you. And now I would like to ask you to listen while we hear Little One's response.

Adult: OK.

Therapist: Little One, how do you respond to Adult?

Little One: I'm afraid Debby will not be able to find any contentment when she feels bad. What would she do when she is lonely, sad, or when things are too hard to handle?

Therapist: That's a good question. Let's listen to Adult's response.

Adult: There has to be a better way to feel content. We have to find something else to do to feel content.

Little One repeated her fear, and the two parts engaged in several minutes of dialogue that resulted in an impasse. Since I already knew that Debby believed in a Higher Power, I decided to take another path to resolution.

Therapist: There is a part of your inner mind, or your subconscious, which is closely connected to your Higher Power. I would like to talk directly to that part of your mind that is most closely connected to God or Higher Power, and ask it to communicate and assist if it is permitted. If you are willing to communicate, please indicate by moving the "yes" finger or by saying the words "I am here."

Part connected to Higher Power: I am here.

Therapist: Thank you for emerging. What name or title shall I call you?

Part connected to Higher Power: Call me Matthew. I'm her Master Guide.

Therapist: Thank you for being here to assist. What suggestions do you have to help us resolve Debby's concerns?

Matthew: This is one of the lessons she's had to learn. She is ready to face this. It is a fear of letting go. Little One has to release the fear.

Therapist: Can you tell Little One exactly what to do?

Matthew: Little One, you can keep the job of contentment, and focus on other ways to help Debby feel contentment. Just release the fear.

Therapist: Little One, how do you respond to Matthew?

Little One: I'm willing to release the fear, but how can I help Debby find other ways to feel content?

138

Matthew: Whenever Debby is sad, have her meditate. Things that will make her content will come to her in meditation.

Therapist: Little One, can you follow Matthew's suggestions?

Little One: Yes. I can do this.

Therapist: Adult, what is your response to Matthew and Little One?

Adult: This feels good! I have no questions.

Therapist: Matthew, do you have any further advice for any of Debby's parts?

Matthew: Call me when you need me.

After confirming the terms of agreement, I integrated the parts and gave suggestions and imagery for Debby's specific benefits that she had previously related to me. When the session was concluded, she was profoundly surprised that the cause was so simple. All these years she overlooked the possibility that contentment was a primary part of the core cause. The other two suspected causes were apparently released in previous therapy sessions.

11.4 Career compromise

Brad volunteered for a session in front of his peers at a parts therapy workshop. Although he was successful in another career, a part of him wanted to jump fulltime into hypnotherapy. He said that another part was holding him back. We pick up the session at Step 5, after the conflicting part emerges. While Brad is not the client's real name, I have used the actual names that the parts provided.

Therapist: Thank you. What name or title shall I call you?

Conflicting Part: Call me Scared.

Therapist: What job do you do for Brad?

Scared: I protect him.

Therapist: How do you protect him?

Scared: I keep him from getting over his head.

Therapist: Why do you feel this is necessary?

Scared: I don't want him to hurt anyone. He wants to help others.

Therapist: Thank you for communicating. Are you willing to listen while I call out another part?

After Scared agreed to listen, I then repeated the first four steps to call out the motivating part: that part that wanted Brad to drop his other career and devote all his professional energy to developing a hypnotherapy career.

Motivating Part: Call me Help.

Therapist: Hello, Help. What job do you do?

Help: I give Brad satisfaction in what he does, a feeling of completeness.

Therapist: How do you respond to Scared?

Help: He can't help people without taking a chance. Scared doesn't want to fail. Brad wants to be his best.

Therapist: How can Brad be his best?

Help: He needs to take a chance.

After thanking Help for speaking and asking him to listen, I then asked Scared to respond.

Scared: There's a lot to lose by switching careers.

Therapist: Help, how do you respond to those concerns?

Help: We've done it before, twenty years ago. Scared needs to give it a chance. I'll protect him.

Therapist: Scared, is that right?

Scared: Yes, he's done it before, but I want Help to come up with a plan—a *safe* plan.

Help: It's hard to come up with a plan when you are coming from fear.

Therapist: Where is this fear coming from?

Help: It's the fear of failure, but it's unreasonable. It's been there all the time.

Scared and Help were unable to resolve their conflict, so I called out that part of the inner mind that had Brad's best wisdom, knowledge, understanding and intelligence. It emerged easily and quickly.

Therapist: Thank you for being here. What words of wisdom do you have?

Self: Follow the heart. Go with what is right. Scared may keep on protecting Brad, but he must move forward and help others. Fear can be kept in balance, but it must not dominate. Brad should go slow, working only part time in hypnotherapy, working two jobs for now.

Both Scared and Help thought that was a good plan, and quickly confirmed their agreement. Then, during the first breakaway practice session, Brad asked another student to find out whether Scared would be willing to take on a new name. It chose the name Farmer. Before studying hypnotherapy, Brad previously considered dropping his sales career in order to buy a farm. Farmer's new job was to help Brad find a way to buy a farm, while Help would establish a plan to help him remain involved in hypnotherapy as well.

11.5 Getting big

Bill felt that he would have more professional credibility if he could lose some of his excess weight. He went up and down like a yo-yo for ten years, always gaining back more weight than he lost. Since we tend to find what we lose, I explained that I do weight management or weight reduction, but not weight loss.

After some additional discussion regarding his inner conflict, he easily entered hypnosis, but his motivating part emerged first, called William. His primary purpose was to motivate Bill to be successful both personally and professionally, but he was getting tired of that part causing him to eat too much.

My second attempt to call out the conflicting part was successful now that William emerged first, because "Billy" was anxious to respond to William.

Billy's job was to protect Bill from bullies, and the world was full of them. When I asked why that was necessary, Billy told me that in grade school he was always short for his age. One time after school a bully beat Billy up when he left the school grounds, sending him home with blood and tears. His mother comforted him and said, "Someday you'll be big, and nobody can pick on you any more!"

Billy took this literally, and determined to keep Bill "big" so that others would be less likely to intimidate him, so he forced Bill to gain weight every time he took it off.

William explained to Billy that size wasn't as important in the adult world unless one were working as a professional athlete, and that he was smart enough to avoid letting others boss him around.

Coming to terms of agreement was relatively easy once Billy understood that Mom meant "adult" rather than "fat" when she told him that someday he would be big. With this new understanding, he changed his job. Instead of making Bill literally big through overeating, he would now protect Bill from anyone trying to manipulate him by warning William. In return, Billy wanted William to take appropriate action if Bill started giving in to inappropriate manipulative demands.

11.6 Big protection

Here is a similar session to the one above, which parallels numerous clients over the years. Judy wanted to get rid of over fifty pounds, which she put on before getting divorced several years earlier. All attempts at weight reduction never got to first base.

The conflicting part called itself Protector. When asked what she protected Judy from, the response was, "Judy was gorgeous in her twenties. Her first husband married her for her looks, and he was a total jerk. My job is to protect her from attracting somebody else who loves her looks instead of loving her for who she is."

Happy (the motivating part) said that Judy would be happier if she went out more often, because her excess weight resulted in very few dates. Protector's response was that the few who did date her were more likely to be right for her. Happy and Protector went back and forth several times with no compromise, until a third part called Wisdom offered to provide both parts with the wisdom to ask the right questions to any man who courted her.

Protector agreed to back off on overeating and let Judy take off *half* of her excess weight in order to improve her looks, and then to let her reduce some more only after getting into a loving relationship. Happy agreed that being slightly overweight was better than carrying her current weight.

11.7 Professional confidence

Chuck knew he was trained competently to sell business services, but experienced a confidence problem. Inner conflicts inhibited his ability to do proper follow-up with prospective clients, so he volunteered for parts therapy. After discussion and induction, two parts easily emerged.

The conflicting part was Critic, whose job was to evaluate Chuck's performance in life and offer constructive criticism. Asking how he did this resulted in a criticism of several of Chuck's shortcomings. He found Chuck to be less than perfect, and punished him for his faults.

The motivating part was called Professional. He knew Chuck's strengths, but was hampered by Critic because he partly agreed with that part's evaluations and criticism, which had become more destructive over the years. Professional wanted Chuck to be his best, but Critic's constant criticism crippled his confidence.

Critic was very verbal in his response to Professional. Asking when he took on the job of evaluating Chuck resulted in a spontaneous regression to childhood, when Chuck's mother told him that a job wasn't worth doing unless you did it right. She also emphasized, "Become perfect as our Father in Heaven is perfect."

A third part called Balance said that perfection in the physical world is often an illusion except when one is dealing with occupations that require perfection, such as accounting. He said, "It is easier to be your best than it is to be perfect, and then to learn from your faults." Balance continued to explain that on one day Chuck's best might be better than his best on another day, depending on how he felt physically or emotionally.

Balance suggested that Critic could now evaluate Chuck's strengths and tell Professional how Chuck could integrate those strengths into his professional activities. Critic agreed, and changed his name to Evaluator. Professional agreed to work in harmony with Evaluator, and Balance agreed to help Chuck live a more balanced life instead of working all the time, so that he would feel better when working.

Chuck's confidence improved greatly in the following months, as did his performance.

11.8 This one is personal

This client was a self-employed person and part-time teacher. His primary concern was to pick up the pieces after seeing an important goal shattered because of trusting the wrong person. A very critical conflicting part, called Judge, drove the client to strive for perfection, yet made him aware of every imperfection on this never-ending quest. He indulged in excessive self-analysis after every class he taught, replaying perceived imperfections instead of focusing on the positive. After an in-depth parts therapy session, Judge agreed that it was OK to simply "be the best you can be". Additionally, this former negative part agreed to take on a new job: putting the important teachings into book form.

Since that session, three books have been written and published. This one on parts therapy is the fourth, because I was the client. One of my former students facilitated a masterful parts therapy session in 1990 to help me deal with my own issues after suffering a major setback. To me, client-centered parts therapy is personal, and profoundly beneficial.

11.9 Sweet tooth

One of my recent hypnotherapy students was a woman with a craving for sweets. She experienced a session with three emerging parts. During the first portion of the parts therapy process (facilitated by another student), Sweet Tooth and Happy ended up coming to terms of agreement regarding food and healthy habits. However, just when integration seemed appropriate, another part called Arts Part emerged. This third part wanted more time for artistic endeavors as well as healthy ones. For example, she was to think about various projects involving the arts. Several weeks later she told me that some very positive benefits resulted from her parts therapy session.

11.10 The rose

In June of 1999, while teaching parts therapy to more than forty professionals in Ireland, something very profound resulted from my second demonstration. I asked for a volunteer who had a simple inner conflict, and Margaret (her real name) came on stage in front of a live audience and a video camera. She couldn't decide whether to buy a new car or keep her old one.

Her motivating part took on her given name, Margaret. The conflicting part, called Careful, told Margaret that she didn't deserve a new car, while the motivating part said that she needed a car that was more dependable. I asked further questions regarding why the conflicting part felt she didn't deserve another car, and what emerged was a feeling of guilt.

Several years earlier, Margaret's mother was killed in a fatal auto accident, and Margaret was driving. What started out as a simple demonstration of parts therapy turned into a profound grief therapy, as I asked the client to do Gestalt role-play with her deceased mother. After many tears, the self-forgiveness provided the necessary release. By break time, I don't believe there was a dry eye in the room.

Three years later, I returned to an audience of 95 therapists in Ireland, and Margaret came up on stage to tell the group about her life-changing experience in 1999. That one session had a ripple effect that helped her both personally and professionally, and she became quite proficient using parts therapy with her clients. She told me that her mother appeared to her in a dream and said, "Give that man a rose."

When Margaret gave me a fresh rose in front of the entire group, I was touched deeply. I pressed it inside the pages of a book in order to preserve it as a memento of an incredible session. Even now it brings tears to my eyes just writing about this, as it was one of most profound public sessions I've ever been privileged to facilitate. Margaret, I still have your rose!

Chapter 12
Potential Pitfalls and Other Concerns

Over the years I've shared both successes and learning experiences with my students. Since childhood, I have endeavored to learn from the mistakes of others in order to avoid their consequences, as an ounce of prevention is worth a pound of cure. My variation on that saying is equally important: *one minute of communication is worth a month of resolution.*

My goal in this chapter is to reveal some potential pitfalls so that you can avoid them when facilitating parts therapy. Knowing the more common ones may result in your being able to help most of the people most of the time rather than helping only some of the people some of the time.

Every potential pitfall discussed in this chapter has claimed its share of professionals and their clients walking the path of parts therapy. While I do not know every possible pit or detour that's out there, I wish to shine the light of perception into the ones that have come to my attention over the years. In my professional opinion, some of them are only minor concerns or shallow pits in the path, resulting in unnecessary detours that may cost nothing more than a few minutes of time. Some pits are deeper, and may result in the client's being farther away from resolution than before the start of attempted therapy. Rather than discuss them in order of importance, let's explore them in alphabetical order.

12.1 Advance explanation not given

It is human nature for us to fear that which we do not understand. The same is true of parts therapy.

Some years back, a client came to me for stress management. During the intake, she informed me that she recently discovered that she had multiple personalities. Although I disclosed to her that I'm neither trained to diagnose (or treat) mental illness, nor to work with multiple personality disorders, I asked her when she was diagnosed. She explained that she came to that opinion about herself several months earlier after several therapy sessions with another therapist. Further discussion revealed that she apparently received a variation of parts therapy without having a proper explanation. The emerging personalities shocked her, but she failed to share her concern with her therapist at the time. Instead, she worried about these new subpersonalities for several months. After hearing my explanation of parts therapy, she wanted me to hypnotize her and call out the same subpersonalities. I quickly learned from the parts that they indeed attained terms of agreement previously with the other therapist, but the lack of proper explanation resulted in unnecessary stress that lasted for several months. She left my office in the state of inner harmony.

The depth of this pit in the path depends on the personality of the client. Some clients may have sufficient trust and rapport with the therapist that they could be quite comfortable with almost any productive therapeutic process employed. Others could become somewhat stressed in the absence of appropriate explanation, just as the woman described above. Personally, I'm unwilling to take any unnecessary chances, so I always provide an advance explanation before employing parts therapy. I recommend that my students do likewise.

If you ever find it necessary to facilitate parts therapy without the advance explanation, please make certain that you still allow sufficient time after concluding the session to provide an explanation that leaves your client feeling comfortable with the experience. A few minutes of simple explanation to a client may prevent months of stress or anxiety.

12.2 *Assuming command and giving orders*

When I first learned parts therapy at the Charles Tebbetts Hypnotism Training Institute, one of my classmates decided that he should assume command of the situation after hearing the two opposing parts speak. He felt that his duty as arbitrator was to determine the best solution himself, and he gave direct suggestions to each part much as a military officer might give orders to enlisted personnel. Within his first few practice sessions he encountered a rebellious part that chose a few choice words before the client (another student) spontaneously emerged from hypnosis. There was no resolution. This pit was deep enough to prevent that student therapist from walking any further along the path of successful parts therapy with his fellow student. Instead, he ended up working with another student in the class.

After presenting my first professional parts therapy workshop, a participant told me that she witnessed a session at another workshop where the facilitator demonstrated a variation of parts therapy, and also gave posthypnotic suggestions prematurely. After allowing each part to present its complaint, he allegedly chose to determine the best solution and then told each part exactly what to do to resolve the client's concern. Although I never learned about the end results, I believe that such an authoritative approach increases the risk of setbacks. I call this *therapist-directed trance work.*

Although I do give direct suggestions during the tenth step, by then I have earned the right to do so. I give them respectfully, as if each part were a person. A therapy style that gives the appearance of disrespect to any of the parts may break rapport and/or cause rebellion. Client-centered parts therapy, in which your client comes up with the solution (even if you help), makes the subconscious more likely to accept direct suggestions after the first nine steps are properly facilitated. If we take shortcuts or talk down to a part, we may encounter subconscious resistance.

In 1983, Charles Tebbetts taught his students to treat each part as though it were a person. Twenty years later, Gordon Emmerson gave the same advice on the printed page in his book on ego-state therapy (2003, page 46). My experience during the intervening years validates the opinion given by these two masters of parts therapy. A little respect and courtesy will go a long way. Remember that it takes only one rebellious part to inhibit resolution of inner conflicts.

Note that in previous writings and workshops, I gave this potential pitfall the label, *Determining the best solution yourself and telling all the parts what to do.*

12.3 Calling out too many parts

This pit is so shallow that both therapist and client might step in it without ever realizing any potential problem. Even Tebbetts sometimes called out numerous parts while facilitating parts therapy.

During my first few years as a hypnotherapist, even while teaching parts therapy at a college, it was common for me to call out several different parts. Certainly, my students witnessed some interesting conversations in the classroom with a hypnotized client allowing several parts to emerge; but these sessions consumed unnecessary amounts of time because parts conversed with little or no relevance to the presenting problem.

Over the years, I learned to call out only those parts that need to communicate in order to help the client attain inner-conflict resolution, which is a more client-centered approach. As emphasized in this book, I initially call out only the conflicting part and the motivating part while helping a client resolve an inner conflict. Only if necessary will I call out additional parts; and only after confirming the terms of agreement will I give an open invitation for the client's other parts to communicate.

Earlier in this book, I discussed the unnecessary detour taken by a participant at a workshop in Ireland, which resulted in a parts party (see 7.1.3, "Calling out a third part", in Chapter 7). While no damage was done, progress was impeded by the presence of several talking parts that had nothing to contribute to the therapy session. Fortunately, the client was a participant in the workshop rather than a client paying more than $100 per hour for the wasted time.

It is quite possible that the only risk to your client is the financial cost of extra therapy time. That being said, some clients might be genuinely interested in knowing about their ego states. Gordon

Emmerson offers a session in which he maps a client's ego states (Emmerson, 2003). In his opinion, clients may feel more empowered knowing about their various ego states; and such awareness benefits both client and therapist alike. If the client knows in advance that numerous parts will be called out, and he/she is willing to invest the extra time and money to learn about these common parts, then be ready for some interesting and lively discussion. I myself might someday be interested in one of Emmerson's maps of my ego states; but it would be done with my permission rather than by therapist-directed trance work.

The bottom line here can be summarized as follows: when the motive is inner-conflict resolution, call out only those parts that are necessary to achieve inner harmony. When the goal is for awareness of the client's various parts (with permission of the client), then go ahead and enjoy facilitating a parts party.

12.4 Creating new parts

Some therapists believe in creating new parts to help a client take on a new job. While this may be considered by some as another path leading to resolution, my own preference would be to ask an existing part to take a new job rather than create another new part to take that job.

According to Emmerson (2003), our parts (or ego states) originate when we are confronted with a frustration or trauma, and have no existing ego state that can respond. While the subconscious seems perfectly capable of creating a new part as a self-defense mechanism, why would the inner mind choose to create another part when an existing part can adequately handle a situation? I believe that we should avoid unnecessary fragmentation of our subconscious.

Although I have stated this opinion publicly in workshops as well as in my classroom, the jury is still out on this issue. An experienced therapist might someday demonstrate an appropriate situation that causes me to reconsider my opinion. Until such time, I will continue to teach my students to follow my steps as they walk down the path of parts therapy and avoid creating new parts.

12.5 *Criticizing a part*

Criticizing someone you meet for the first time is not the best way to win friends and influence people, and the same is true for ego parts. They tend to resist or resent criticism. While you might know your client fairly well, treat each part as you would if meeting someone for the first time. Break rapport with a part, and you break rapport with the subconscious. Your client could easily emerge from trance before you realize what is happening.

Even if the client remains in hypnosis, your job as a mediator is far easier if all the participating parts feel comfortable with you. Who among us feels comfortable around someone who criticizes us? Someone who dishes out frequent criticism often puts others on the defensive. A part that feels it is on the defensive is less likely to be amicable, and could become totally uncooperative.

Occasionally, a therapist might unintentionally criticize or offend a part. If that happens, we should simply apologize just as we might with a person. Once rapport is regained, then continue with whatever step is appropriate in the parts therapy process. Remember that maintaining rapport is easier than rebuilding rapport that was lost.

12.6 *Freezing or immobilizing a part*

A close personal friend of mine, who also studied hypnotherapy under Tebbetts, reported an unusual case to me. One of his former classmates worked with a woman whose parts apparently did not respond very well to the parts therapy process. In frustration, the therapist "froze" several parts into statues because they did not want to take on a new job for the client. The resulting stress made the woman worse off than before, and my friend spent two lengthy sessions undoing the damage done by his former classmate. If you are in doubt as to how to proceed during a parts therapy process, ask the parts to agree to continue at another appropriate time and place. Then integrate, awaken, and seek help or refer!

12.7 Getting sidetracked

This almost seems too obvious to mention, but it is easy to get side-tracked and forget that parts were called out when a spontaneous regression occurs, or when giving hypnotic suggestions during the tenth step. While giving posthypnotic suggestions, we should remember whether we are giving suggestions to an individual part, or to the entire person (all the parts of the whole).

Once, when I experienced parts therapy for a personal issue, the therapist got sidetracked into a hypnotic regression. She awakened me after facilitating the regression properly. After spending the next day thinking about the regression almost every waking minute, I reflected back on the session and realized that she forgot to complete the parts therapy process and integrate my parts. Her oversight resulted in my being greatly distracted at work until I corrected the situation with a simple autosuggestion during a brief self-hypnotic meditation. I gave myself the idea that my finger would move when my parts were properly integrated. Even if I had not known what to do, I don't believe any permanent damage would have resulted; but most likely I might have experienced several days of strange thoughts before my mind integrated itself. (It turned out that the therapist had not received actual training in parts therapy, but had only read about it in *Miracles on Demand* by Tebbetts.)

Also, a friend of mine was only in a light trance when a counselor used *voice dialogue*, a variation of parts therapy. My friend felt his conscious mind analyzing so much that, after several minutes into the voice dialogue technique, he exclaimed, "This isn't working!" Since both he and the therapist falsely assumed that no hypnosis took place, there was no integration process. This left him disoriented for a couple of days, because his "parts" had actually emerged during the light hypnotic state; and it took two days for his mind to gradually integrate by itself.

12.8 Multiple personality disorder

I will not knowingly work with someone who has multiple personalities without supervision from a psychotherapist or psychologist trained and experienced in working with clients with MPD (also known as DID, for dissociative identity disorder).

That being said, I will always remember a lengthy conversation with a hypnotherapist at an international hypnotherapy convention years ago. She told me that she was a "recovered MPD". As a child, she almost worshipped her father, who was a minister. When she bloomed into adulthood in her teens, her father raped her. Her primary personality could not handle the trauma of her father shattering her image of him, so another part of her walled itself off from the primary personality in order to prevent her from killing herself. What once was a part whose job was to protect her took that job one step farther by walling itself off totally like a separate personality. That second personality hated men, and was rebellious; but it protected the primary personality by making sure no memories leaked over. When Dad continued to molest her, the second personality got tired of the pain—and another part became a third personality. The third personality realized that sex was not painful if it was enjoyed, so it protected the rebellious part as well as the primary part. Later, a fourth personality formed.

Eventually, she realized that something was happening during the memory blackout periods, and sought help. A psychiatrist spent many months studying her as the subject of scientific study. A psychologist then counseled her on how to cope with being an MPD. That was not good enough for her, and she eventually found a psychologist who was also trained in one of the variations of parts therapy. Through the combination of hypnotic regression therapy and parts therapy, he helped her integrate the personalities. The woman who spoke with me said, "I am the integrated person, and I can remember my parts becoming separate personalities, because it was the only way for me to cope with what happened to me." Her own recovery through parts therapy and hypnosis resulted in her becoming a certified hypnotherapist.

Several years later, I met another hypnotherapist who claimed that she had seven personalities most of her life. She said five were already integrated through the combination of regression and parts therapy, and she had two more left to integrate. Upon hearing her taped sessions, she said that each subsequent personality knew of the ones before, but not the ones that split off afterwards. Apparently personality #7 knew of all the others. At a conscious level, she had conscious awareness only of the ones already integrated. It was her opinion that her personalities were originally parts that walled themselves off during childhood trauma.

While I do not claim to be an expert by any stretch of the imagination in MPD, somehow the experiences of these two hypnotherapists seem very relevant to include in this book. My recommendation is that if you have a client who gives you reason to suspect MPD, consider either referring the client to another professional or get the client's written permission for you to consult with a professional trained and experienced with clients who have multiple personalities.

That being said, a psychotherapist took my hypnosis course several years ago in order to learn parts therapy. His experience included working with MPD cases. He felt that many therapists taught the client with multiple personalities simply to live with their condition and cope with it. (Others studied the client as an object of scientific study.) It was his opinion that many of these people could be helped through the combination of counseling and hypnotherapy, combining regression therapy with parts therapy.

In my opinion, the use of hypnotic parts therapy to help people with multiple personality disorder is still a wide-open field that requires much more research and experimentation. However, if you are a hypnotherapist without the background in counseling or psychology, do both yourself and your clients a favor: either seek out a competent professional who is trained and experienced with the MPD to collaborate with your work, or refer the client to an appropriate professional.

If you are already experienced in working with MPD clients, you might consider investing in Emmerson's *Ego State Therapy* (2003), and pay close attention to his comments in the fourth chapter of his excellent book.

12.9 Possible or alleged entities

More than once I've observed facilitators attempting to destroy a rebellious or negative part. On numerous occasions over the years, students and experienced hypnotherapists alike have reported witnessing similar occurrences at various classes and workshops. Some therapists assume that an uncooperative part is an entity that must be cast out or sent into the Light. In my opinion, this practice is questionable at best, and very risky whenever initiated by the facilitator without being requested by the client. The practice of looking for parts (or entities) to cast out may also be considered inappropriate leading.

Those therapists who practice what they call "spiritual hypnotherapy" might immediately be concerned by my above comments in this very lengthy chapter section, so let me provide an in-depth discussion of what may be the most controversial topic of this entire book.

Before discussing the risks of therapist-directed entity release, let's look at two possible reasons for considering the release of an alleged entity: (a) a part claims to be an entity, or (b) the client requests entity release. There are still some potential pits.

12.9.1 What if the part claims to be an entity?

So what happens when a negative part claims that it is an entity? Is it really a foul spirit, or is it simply a figment of the client's imagination?

Emmerson considers such to be a malevolent state, while Hal and Sidra Stone use the label of *disowned part*. William Baldwin, author of several books, including *Spirit Releasement Therapy* (1995), considers them to be entities that must be released through some sort of process that resembles an exorcism. Many religious people will immediately agree with Baldwin and assume that such a part would indeed be a demonic or negative entity, as do some hypnotherapists and psychotherapists. We can debate this question for many years and still have opposing opinions within both the scientific community and the hypnotherapy profession.

Rather than engaging in such a no-win debate or taking a firm position on either side, my goal is to find a way for my client to be free and empowered. Although I do not go looking for entities, when a part claims to be one, my recommendation is that we deal with what emerges. I proceed as though the part truthfully identified itself as an entity. Unlike those who specialize in entity release and write hundreds of pages describing various exorcism techniques, my approach remains simple and client-centered.

First, I do make one assumption that has held true so far for over twenty years. If a part claims to be an entity, the client believes in a Higher Power at some level of consciousness. Thus, I endeavor to call out that part of my client that has the closest connection to God or his/her Higher Power. After taking a deep breath myself and saying a quick silent prayer, I say:

There is a part of you that is most closely connected to God [or Higher Power]. **That part has access to wisdom that can provide great benefit right now. It is important for** [client name] **that I speak with that part now. If it is permitted, please say the words "I am here" or move the yes finger.**

If the client previously disclosed that he/she believes in a Higher Self, Christ, or the Holy Spirit, then I attempt to call out the Higher Self or the Holy Spirit.

It is important for [client name] **that I speak with the Higher Self** [or Holy Spirit]. **That part has access to wisdom that can provide great benefit right now. If it is permitted, please say the words "I am here" or move the yes finger.**

Once that part emerges, I thank it for emerging, and ask about its name or title.

If the part does not emerge, my second request is to communicate directly with the client's Higher Power. With persistence (as of the writing of this book), I have always succeeded in calling out a part that displayed some spiritual authority with my client.

My first response to the Higher Power part is to thank it for being here and ask about its name or title just as with any part. If I have any question about whether this part truly is the Inner Strength part (or Higher Power etc.), I ask:

Do you serve the Light?

Once I'm satisfied that I have a Godlike part, I proceed with:

[Client name] **has a part that claims to be** [entity name or title]. **Please tell us how to proceed.**

From here I simply ask the Higher Power (Higher Self etc.) part to give me step-by-step instructions on how to deal with the alleged entity. Sometimes it is simply a disowned part that needs a new and productive job, as well as acceptance by the client and his/her other parts. Occasionally Higher Power identifies it as an entity, and asks me to dismiss it. Such dismissal almost always involves first asking the client if he/she wishes to release the alleged entity.

Frequently I'm instructed to call on the name of Jesus before dismissing the part in his name. Sometimes, Higher Power tells the client to invite an archangel (Michael or Gabriel) to assist, or some other "ascended master." On one occasion a client was instructed to invite both Buddha and Christ. Occasionally, the client asks a Higher Power to escort the alleged entity away. Often it is released into the Light, and goes on its own when told to do so or when escorted. Some call it exorcism.

Sometimes, an alleged entity resists my calling out a Higher Power by refusing to shut up. Several years ago a part claiming to be a lost soul said, "You have no power over me!"

My immediate response was, "You're right! I don't have any power over you; but someone else does." Before I could say anything more, the entity part started calling me four-letter words. Since I already knew my client believed in Christ, I interrupted with, "By the name and power of Christ, I command you to shut up." In a natural voice, my client thanked me just as though he were a third-party observer to this drama. The client's Higher Power then provided instructions on how to proceed. According to my client, Jesus escorted this particular entity to a black hole to be imprisoned for several centuries. Was this real or imagined? Was it an exorcism, or a confabulation? This is anyone's guess. The point is that my opinion does not matter, because the client was empowered.

12.9.2 What if the client wants a part dismissed?

On rare occasions, the client might initiate the request to have an alleged entity or negative part dismissed. The request may come from the client before hypnosis, or from one of the parts during hypnosis.

Even when the client asks me in advance of the session to assist in releasing an alleged entity or earthbound soul, I do not assume. Instead, I call out the client's Higher Power and ask for assistance. Here is what I say to the Higher Power:

[Client name] **believes that there is an entity** [or earthbound soul etc.] **influencing him/her. Would you please provide some words of wisdom on how to proceed?**

Again (as mentioned above) I follow the instructions. Occasionally, the motivating part wants an uncooperative conflicting part dismissed (or vice versa). Usually, this results from a lack of trust between the two parts in conflict. I ignore the request, and continue right on in my attempts to negotiate terms of agreement. Often, the previously uncooperative part will end up taking on a new job. Frequently (but not always), I find it necessary to call out a third part to assist in the mediation when this occurs.

If we call out additional parts, and they all want the uncooperative part dismissed, we have another concern. For years, I taught my students that they should *never* take it upon their own initiative to cast out a part unless all the other parts unanimously wanted it dismissed. This opinion was slightly modified after I had worked with a client who had two parts engaging in very vocal conflict and unable to come to terms of agreement. When I called out the client's Higher Self, it quickly informed me that the conflicting part was a negative entity, and that I should send it into the Light. Without trying to determine whether said entity was real or imagined, I followed the instructions of Higher Self. Even then, the part was dismissed but not destroyed, although we could certainly debate that outcome based on whether it was a negative part or a real entity. We may also speculate whether or not it was really an exorcism, or simply a subconscious perception of releasing a negative energy through suggestion and imagery. The successful outcome was more important than knowing whether or not the alleged entity was real.

Note that, once the Higher Power part speaks, I still avoid asking a leading question. Rather than ask if the part is an entity or whatever, I ask,

What words of wisdom do you have regarding [part name or Client name]?

I then follow the instructions given by the Higher Power part.

12.9.3 The therapist initiates the decision

Let me begin this lengthy subsection by reviewing some very important comments made earlier.

A deeply hypnotized client is *in rapport* with the hypnotist. If the level of trance is deep enough, that person may have an emotional desire to please the hypnotist, and provide whatever answers are expected.

When uninformed hypnotists or psychotherapists use hypnotic regression to look for past abuse, they may often find it where it never existed, and this results in false memories. Likewise, when hypnotists or psychotherapists use hypnosis or variations of parts therapy to look for entities, the subconscious is perfectly capable of having a part put on a convincing show. In other words, "seek and you shall find" applies here, even if the "entity" is found only in the imagination of both client and therapist alike. In other words, confabulation may occur if a deeply hypnotized client with an emerging part called Guilty hears a question such as, "Is Guilty really an influencing or possession entity? If so, move the yes finger."

I realize that many people would rather blame the devil instead of taking responsibility for their own actions; so it is very easy for an unsuspecting client to have a part pretend to be a negative entity to take the blame away from the other parts.

During the early 1990s, I witnessed a workshop facilitator doing exactly what I described two paragraphs above (asking a leading question about an entity). Afterwards, I confronted him privately and asked him how often he got a yes answer to such a question. As I suspected, he admitted that he always got an affirmative response. We had some lengthy words about the consequences of inappropriate leading. To his credit, he agreed with me and promised to change his methods.

Years ago, I knew a woman who was abused by both her father and her first husband. An ordained minister with a doctorate in psychology treated her with parts therapy in front of a group of students, and he rebuked a rebellious part that talked back to him. He asserted his authority and commanded the part to be consumed by the "ever-consuming flame of Christ". According to a witness, that part talked back with some rather vulgar language before the session ended without resolution. Afterwards, this same woman refused to work with a male therapist as a direct result of that experience.

In the mid-1990s, while attending a national hypnosis convention, I enjoyed a snack in the hotel lobby. Meanwhile, a hypnosis instructor approached and asked if he could join me and get something off of his chest. He had just walked out of a workshop on "spiritual hypnosis" that had a filled room. Before knowing what would happen, he volunteered to be hypnotized in front of the audience, only to have the facilitator call out an alleged entity from him and do an exorcism. It was his strong personal opinion that his subconscious fantasized the entity in order to please the facilitator. Also, he held the strong professional opinion that such inappropriate leading could easily cause confabulation of such an entity. I voiced my agreement. In short, if you go looking for entities, you shall surely find them, whether or not they are real or imagined.

Here are my primary concerns regarding therapist-directed entity release:

- What are the possible consequences of residual guilt for a client believing that such an "entity" influenced them in the first place?
- What if a part that is mistaken for an entity is really a part that could take on a more productive job?
- What if the release of the alleged entity creates guilt that escalates into a traumatic experience?
- What are the legal concerns for therapist-directed release of alleged entities?

Let me address the first three concerns with the following example. Before the twentieth century drew to a close, a very competent hypnotherapist (and personal friend) asked me to facilitate a session for professional confidence. Some months earlier he attended a presentation on "spiritual hypnosis" at a national hypnosis convention, and volunteered to be hypnotized in front of his peers. One of his parts was allegedly identified as a negative entity by the presenter, and exorcised in front of the group. His feeling of guilt increased during the weeks that followed, taking his confidence and private practice downhill. I called out his Higher Power, who quickly claimed that he never had a negative entity in the first place, and stated that said entity was projected into him by the expectations of the facilitator at that workshop. The part that was crippled by guilt and sent into hiding at the workshop was, in reality, a very important part that contributed to my friend's professional confidence. With the help of Higher Power, "Confidence" came out of hiding and empowered him to be his best, and probably saved his career. I believe that the original workshop facilitator is lucky that my friend chose the path of forgiveness rather than the path of litigation. Initiating an entity release work may make a therapist vulnerable to legal action, especially with a client who is not as forgiving.

As should be evident by now, I strongly discourage any therapist from ever initiating the decision to facilitate a hypnotic entity release. Also, I believe that it is imperative for us to avoid bringing up the subject of entities, whether before or during hypnosis.

12.10 Skipping steps

The potential risk of skipping steps may vary anywhere from non-existent to severe. This depends on the combination of the client's personality, the presenting problem, the parts involved in the process, and which step(s) the therapist omits. In my earlier years of teaching, I became concerned when some of my students encountered problems as a result of skipping one or more of the steps. The mild problems were sessions that took a little more time and determination from therapist and client alike for all participating parts to attain terms of agreement. Occasionally, a student who skipped a step failed to obtain resolution, and subsequent sessions were necessary.

By the late 1990s, role-play exercises in the classroom helped to minimize this concern, and I also utilize this valuable learning tool in my workshops. I pretend to be a client in hypnosis with an inner conflict. Meanwhile, students (or workshop participants) take turns playing the role of therapist. This method of teaching enhances learning in a safe and supervised environment. If a student skips a step (or walks into another pitfall described in this chapter), I can then respond in a way that might happen in an actual session. Students witness potential problems in role-play without having to deal with real consequences. Positive feedback validates this as an excellent method of teaching parts therapy, and it helps students get accustomed to following all eleven steps.

A few hypnotherapists facilitate parts therapy without employing all of the steps presented in this book. Even though many of their sessions are successful, I believe that following the entire eleven-step process will increase the probability of lasting success.

12.11 Taking sides with the dominant part

Here is another important difference between my work and the earlier work of my former mentor, mentioned in Chapter 2, Section 2.2 ("Important updates"). As mentioned in the second chapter, Charles Tebbetts taught his students to side in with the dominant part, and to persuade the conflicting part to change. He was a debate champion in high school, and enjoyed debating with the various parts of his clients. This plan is risky for most of us, however, as a part can easily be offended by such debate.

Also, as we saw in that same section of Chapter 2, Charlie wanted his students to act like an arbitrator. Instead, I teach my students to take on the role of mediator. Much more can be accomplished through good listening and remaining objective, especially when we build and maintain rapport with all the parts. If one part feels as though you are taking sides with another part, you can kiss rapport goodbye. I cannot overestimate the importance of maintaining rapport throughout the entire parts therapy process. If you break rapport with a "part" by failing to be a good listener while it presents its case, your role as a facilitator becomes difficult if not impossible.

Let's remember my former student who learned this lesson the hard way after taking sides with the dominant part. (See the same section of Chapter 2 again for details.) His client would not re-enter hypnosis, even after several attempts, until after the therapist pologized to the offended part. This demonstrates that our parts are listening even when we are fully conscious.

12.12 Other concerns

Although other potential pitfalls may exist, I discussed the most common ones in this chapter. Those most likely to fall into a pitfall are therapists who take short cuts with either the hypnotic process or with the parts therapy process. This often happens as a result of inadequate hypnosis training.

Some psychotherapists make the mistake of assuming that a background in counseling is an acceptable substitute for competent hypnosis training, and they may be vulnerable to facilitating therapist-directed trance work. Regardless of credentials, those who practice therapist-directed trance work are tempted to project their own expectations into the client, increasing the risk of confabulation. This can be especially true for a mental health counselor who is trained to diagnose and form preconceived opinions on the cause(s) of a client's problem. It is equally true for a psychic who believes that his or her "psychic gifts" make it acceptable to use the trance to "prove" to the client the validity of the preconceived intuitive opinion.

I believe that a thorough training in the art of hypnosis is an important prerequisite for anyone facilitating client-centered parts therapy, even those with counseling experience. Personally, when I'm the client, I prefer working with a competently trained hypnotherapist without a counseling background to working with an experienced psychotherapist who has little or no training in hypnosis. Here is my recommendation to psychotherapists or anyone wishing to facilitate parts therapy: *master the art of hypnosis first*.

Now let's go where few have gone before: into the undiscovered country of the inner mind.

Chapter 13
New Frontiers
The Undiscovered Country

New frontiers of possibility exist in the undiscovered country of the subconscious, especially regarding our potential connection to a Higher Power. These are the voyages of the inner mind, to seek out new ideas, and to boldly go where few have gone before.

On numerous occasions over the years, I've used an application of parts therapy to access that part of the inner mind that is most closely connected to God, or the client's perception of Higher Power. Frequently the client obtains deeply encouraging insights, along with important information regarding the purpose in life. Whether or not one believes in God or a Higher Power, the subconscious (or unconscious) contains access to an inner wisdom that sometimes far surpasses that of ordinary consciousness.

Before I share my own journeys, let me mention that I'm not alone in this discovery.

13.1 Experts visit new frontiers

Other experts in variations of parts therapy have also discovered spiritual parts. Consider the words of the following professionals, whose books are available in libraries and bookstores in many different countries.

Emmerson discusses the "Inner Strength" part in the very first chapter of his book *Ego State Therapy* (2003). This ego state may refer to itself as "Higher Self" or "spiritual self". Emmerson states that everyone appears to have an inner strength state.

John Rowan devoted an entire chapter to this same topic in his book, *Discover Your Subpersonalities* (1993). On page 173, he writes: "Amazing insight can come from such parts of ourselves. When such a voice is contacted, a strong empowerment may take place. We are beginning to connect to inner sources of strength and wisdom."

Rowan goes on to warn us not to confuse this spiritual energy with an "inner pusher". He provides some valuable insight on how to tell the difference. The pusher may be judgmental, opinioned, critical, and controlling or defensive etc. The Higher Self is compassionate, loving, wise, forgiving, and nurturing or peaceful etc.

Hal and Sidra Stone, recognized pioneers of voice dialogue, also devoted an entire chapter to spiritual selves in *Embracing Our Selves* (1989). On pages 218–19 they write:

> In Voice Dialogue, we can contact another self—a self that can open us to our spiritual selves. This self is more concerned with being than with doing. When we experience this "being" energy, there is no goal and no task …

They go on to mention that the client is in a meditative state. Like Rowan, they describe the spiritual energy as nonjudgmental and uplifting. However, they believe that voice dialogue can work with spiritual energies only to a limited extent. This leaves a very important question to consider: would deeper trance states make a difference with some of their observations? My professional opinion is a resounding yes.

The remaining pages of this book reveal some results obtained during deep hypnosis in past sessions. They provide some serious food for thought, or perhaps I should say *food for the soul*.

13.2 Seeking resolution from a spiritual part

Let's first consider the application of parts therapy that differs from the one presented in this book. Rather than calling out two parts in conflict, my first choice is to call out the part that is most closely connected to God or the client's perception of Higher Power.

Again, my first objective after the hypnotic induction is to get the client as deep as possible. The lighter the trance state, the greater the risk of interference from either the conscious mind or a part connected with the ego. On a recent occasion where the client was not deep enough, a part emerged that pretended to be a spiritual part. Within just a few minutes, the criticism and self-doubt spewing from my client's mouth made it obvious that I was not talking to a spiritual part. The session became a traditional parts therapy session even though the client initially requested to contact his Higher Power.

Now let's take our first step into the undiscovered country of the inner mind.

13.2.1 The Road

Dan volunteered at a taped workshop to let me demonstrate how to call out the Higher Power in order to be better able to stay on what he termed "The Road". He felt that doing hypnotherapy full time was the road that was intended for him, and he wanted to find the confidence to leave his other source of income behind. Dan asked me to call out his Higher Self in order to gain access to a greater wisdom.

Before the session I explained to Dan (and the entire audience) that we can confabulate (or fantasize) a "Higher Self" part if we go into hypnosis with a preconceived idea of what we want to hear. I emphasized the importance of participating in a session like this with an open mind, free of preconceived opinions. Also it is imperative that both the facilitator and the client set aside any preconceived opinions, otherwise those opinions could taint the trance and influence the outcome.

The part that emerged asked me to call it Higher Self, and gave Dan advice to take small steps. Higher Self also told him to stay at his day job a little longer, and to seek advice from a colleague. After the session, Dan told the group, "This seems like a reasonable compromise to my inner conflict—and it was so easy!"

13.2.2 *Light for the life path*

This session was surprisingly short. Shirley wanted advice from her Higher Power regarding her current life path. That part most closely connected with God told me to call it Light.

When I told Light that Shirley requested advice regarding her life path, Light told her to let go of control. Shirley could best accomplish this by *being* love, and by trusting herself more. Light told her to give up the need to control, and surrender it to her Higher Power. I asked for further clarification, and Light told her to sit back and hang on for a real ride. More information would be revealed to her when appropriate. Light also told her that she knows more than she thinks, and ended the message by telling her to relax and stop trying so hard.

Shirley apparently related very well to this information. Enough was resolved to enable her to cancel a private session that she had previously scheduled to take place after the workshop. I wish her well.

13.2.3 *Awareness of life path*

Randy worked at a job he didn't like. In addition to vocational concerns, he wanted to know more about his life path. These were the two primary questions he wanted me to ask: (1) Should Randy stay at his present job?; (2) What is Randy's primary life purpose? His Higher Power requested to be called Holy Spirit.

When Holy Spirit responded to the first question, Randy received advice to remain at his current job while considering other avenues of employment. He also had the option of consulting a vocational counselor, but was reminded to make his own decisions rather than give away his power of choice.

The response to Randy's second question provided some answers with additional questions left unanswered. Holy Spirit told him that he was to learn how to love, and to love the learning process enough to be willing to teach others. When asked when and how he would teach others, Holy Spirit said, "It will be revealed in due time, at the appropriate time and place. Randy needs to trust God, and accept his God-given intuition, and balance it with wisdom rather than emotion."

Randy understood the last statement perfectly, but left with curiosity regarding the comments about his teaching others, as he lived alone. He later realized that he could teach his children spiritual concepts during their weekend visits, and engage in spiritual discussions when others expressed an interest.

13.2.4 Divine guidance

Mary attended a parts therapy workshop and requested a private session with me. She agreed to share her session in this book in hopes that her experience may help others.

Her primary concern involved being angry or sad whenever she felt the need to meet expectations, whether those demands were placed on her by others or by her own conscious mind. A part of her wanted to rebel at many expectations. She desired to accomplish more goals and feel a better sense of self-worth.

Although I attempted to call out the conflicting part first, I soon realized that the motivating part emerged instead. Without reading ahead, see if you can determine when I first realized that it was the motivating part. We pick up the session as I go from Step 4 to Step 5.

Therapist: Thank you for communicating. What name or title shall I call you?

Alleged Conflicting part: Call me Alone.

Therapist: Hello, Alone. What job do you do for Mary?

Alone: Protection—from hurt and disappointment.

Therapist: How do you accomplish this?

Alone: I make her meet other people's expectations.

Therapist: Why do you do that?

Alone: To get attention—but I'm just a little tired of it. I'd rather be alone, away from the demands of others. That feels better than having them be disappointed when I fail to meet their expectations.

Therapist: Thank you for communicating. Are you willing to listen while I call out another part?

Alone: Yes.

At this point, I make a second attempt to call out the conflicting part. If the conflicting part hesitates when first called, the motivating part may emerge first because the desire to change is strong. Although Alone's job (protection) is frequently done by a conflicting part, the answer to my second question ("How do you accomplish this?") made me realize which part emerged first. We now resume the session after the conflicting part emerges.

Therapist: Thank you for speaking. What name or title shall I call you?

Conflicting part: Because.

Therapist: Hi, Because. What job do you do for Mary?

Because: My job is to ask questions. I want reasons before submitting to the demands of others.

Therapist: How do you do this?

Because: I ask questions in my mind.

Therapist: Why is it necessary to ask questions?

Because: Her parents always questioned what she did. Also, because I was always doubted, I torture myself with questions.

Therapist: How do you respond to Alone?

Alone complained about Mary's efforts to meet other people's demands, and said that Mary would not feel alone if she learned to love herself. The additional dialogue between the two parts failed to result in terms of agreement, so I called out that part of Mary most closely connected to her Higher Power. (Note that I have quotations around "Because" in the following exchange merely for clarification that it was the name of a part.)

Therapist: Thank you for being here. What name or title shall I call you?

Higher Power: Call me Divine Guidance.

Therapist: Hello, Divine Guidance. What words of wisdom do you have for Mary and her parts?

Divine Guidance: "Because" needs to be more trusting, and Alone needs to know she has all the knowledge. "Because" does not choose to trust, and Alone is afraid to trust. She must let the hurt go.

Therapist: How can she let the hurt go?

Divine Guidance: By trusting in me. "Because" and Alone need to trust me, and this will help Mary to let go and trust the process. Mary needs to commit to a time of trust. She needs to let the other stuff go and give it time to work. She needs to get back to meditation and go back to the self-hypnosis tapes.

Therapist: What about meeting the expectations of others?

Divine Guidance: Give it up. She must make her own choices in life.

Therapist: Can you clarify? How does this relate to her life purpose?

Divine Guidance: Mary, the Universe wants to stop dragging you. Trust that there is a purpose. The need to ask questions must decrease, and trust needs to increase. Live in your heart instead of your head. This does not have to be hard. Let go, and let it happen.

Therapist: Do you have any additional word of wisdom for Mary?

Divine Guidance: She does not trust herself, nor does she trust her intuition. Mary needs to realize that she had already done more than others give her credit for.

Both parts accepted the advice from Divine Guidance, and agreed to work together. After integration, I gave Mary suggestions to use the advice from Divine Guidance for her highest and best good, and to combine her intuition with her best wisdom, knowledge, intelligence, experience and training. I also suggested that she enjoy a greater self-empowerment than ever before.

We may have varied opinions regarding the true identity of Divine Guidance. Does our opinion really matter regarding whether Divine Guidance was a part of Mary, or the essence of God speaking through a part? Your guess is a good as mine. More important than opinions is the fact that Mary benefited from the session. Several weeks later she sent me the following:

> Some after therapy comments ... I took your notes and carefully folded them and put them into an envelope. I wanted to give some time to the event and see how I felt without diving into the actual particulars of the session. I've been fine; no questioning of much anymore. Divine Guidance won the day. I don't allow myself to get upset when others pull my strings (well, I'm not perfect, but much, much better). I seem to be into the flow much more. So thank you for such profound work. I hope I can help someone else as much as you have helped me ... I'm really looking forward to the release of your book. Thank you again for the session and the workshop.
>
> Kind regards and blessings, Mary

13.3 Unresolved past grief

Let's now enter a frontier that some therapists are already exploring: *unresolved past grief*. Sometimes this may happen during a routine parts therapy session, as evidenced by, Section 11.10, "The rose", in Chapter 11. However, over the years I have frequently facilitated sessions where the specific goal was to help clients find resolution with unresolved past grief that frequently goes clear back to childhood. This often happens outside of parts therapy, in a form of Gestalt role-play with the departed loved one. There are two ways to facilitate hypnotic grief therapy. Let's discuss both.

13.3.1 Resolution with hypnotic regression

The obvious way is through hypnotic regression therapy, by taking the client back in time to visit with the late loved one while he or she was still alive. As with traditional hypnotic regression, I use Gestalt role-play for the client to dialogue with the person he/she needs to release. One such session occurred with a student in my classroom several years ago. She never came to terms with the loss of a grandparent during childhood, who died before she could say goodbye. I regressed her to childhood, and had her imagine being able to say her last goodbye. By the time the session ended, there was not a dry eye in the classroom.

A couple of years later, one of my students asked me to help him deal with the loss of his brother, killed in a bicycling accident during childhood. The letter he sent me appeared in *The Art of Hypnotherapy* with his permission:

> Thank you so very much for the recent work you've done for me in the grief session. I feel I have been able to set at rest my sorrow for not being able to have said goodbye to my younger brother and my father at the time of their deaths. I especially appreciate your sensitivity concerning my religious beliefs, or spiritual preferences. I really felt a burden lifted from my mind. I now feel completely at peace with my brother and my father.

13.3.2 Gestalt role-play in a sacred place

The second method is to guide the client to his or her sacred place, and suggest that the client may now communicate directly to his or her late relative etc. I incorporate Gestalt role-play between the client and the soul (or Higher Self) of the departed loved one. We can debate whether or not the client actually is speaking to the loved one, or to a figment of his/her imagination. In my opinion, the scientific minds can spend their time and money exploring the answer to that question, while those who master the art of hypnosis continue to help people heal themselves emotionally through the benefits of such techniques.

Did you notice my wording in the last sentence of the above paragraph? I believe that *the client is the one who heals himself or herself* emotionally from unresolved grief. The therapist only facilitates the process by guiding the client into deep hypnosis, and by asking the right questions. When the client has the opportunity to say goodbye, even if only in fantasy, this often results in some profound emotional healing as well as greater self-empowerment.

This type of profound grief-therapy session took place in front of a live audience overseas before the dawn of the twenty-first century. Let's discuss that remarkable session now.

13.3.3 The diamond

Betty's parents got divorced when she was a child, and she rarely saw her father afterwards. He then passed on before her 23rd birthday, further complicating her emotional state of mind. Although she was a therapist herself, no amount of conscious logic was ever able to help her overcome her sense of guilt for not being present when her father died. She carried her unresolved grief into her middle age. After a brief discussion in front of other therapists and a videotape recorder, I hypnotized her deeply. Then, before beginning the Gestalt role-play, I asked her Higher Power to assist her through the process.

When Betty's father appeared in her sacred place, he told her to remember the diamond, as it would remind her of the love he felt for her. In addition, it would remind Betty of her own important qualities. She still had difficulty forgiving herself, until her father told her that he had *always forgiven her* for not being there at his passing. Betty started crying.

Her father told her that he was the one who gave her the diamond that she appreciated, and that it should remind her of his love. He also told her to consider the diamond as a metaphor to remind her of other important character qualities she displayed, and that she needed to release him and get on with her life. The diamond opened the door for her to appreciate all the wonderful qualities of herself as well as of the diamond: strong, powerful, clear, and reflecting the light. Her father also told her to be the best that she could be.

I then asked how this information could best benefit Betty in the here and now. The response was, "I never attributed the diamond to my father. He gave it to me! It's what he passed on to me." She went on to admit that it was time to release him.

One of the most profound statements came when she spoke in the voice of her father: "Where I'm speaking from, there is nothing but love." He went on to tell Betty that he loved her, and that she should love him. He said, "That's all there needs to be."

He also told her to tell others about the diamond. She responded by saying that she now felt *complete*. One of my posthypnotic sugges-tions was, "You feel a greater inner peace than you've ever known before ..." As the session progressed, the outside rain was followed by sunshine that broke through at the same time my client attained her resolution. Everyone in the room noticed this rather strange coincidence, and the camcorder picked up someone's comment afterwards about the timing of the sunshine.

After the session, Betty told the audience that she had never attrib-uted the diamond to her father before. She also said, "The diamond makes me feel complete." She praised her instructor (my sponsor for that workshop) and also added, "I will never be the same person again. I will be a far better person than I've ever been before."

Now let's explore another session that ventures into realms of the soul or spirit. It involves more than simple grief therapy. We will explore this one in depth.

13.4 Healing the soul

Carol had several concerns, including unresolved grief that was with her for years. Two parts emerging earlier called themselves Driver and Sadness. Driver provided an ambitious energy and drive that helped Carol accomplish much, but often without listening to any input from the other parts. Sadness felt deep sorrow at life's setbacks and unexpected disappointments. Sadness also felt sad that Driver never listened to her. A third part, Guidance, tried to provide guidance to Carol's life, but Driver also turned a deaf ear to Guidance as well as to Sadness. The parts were unable to attain resolution, so I called out the part of Carol's inner mind that was most closely connected to God. We pick up the session right after the Higher Power part asked to be called Goddess.

Therapist: Hello, Goddess. What words of wisdom do you have for Carol?

Goddess: It is time to heal. I've come to wrap you in love and light, tranquility and peace. It is time for this to come to the microcosm of the larger macrocosm of her. She knows this concept; she lives it. This is what they have always wanted. Driver and Sadness must surrender, and resolve their anger. If what Driver says is true, her greatest desire is to propel Carol into her spiritual path. It is time to relinquish control, and trust God.

Therapist: Driver, how do you respond to Goddess?

Driver: I know you're right.

Therapist: What will it take for you to follow the advice of Goddess?

Driver: I want Carol to have financial security—money to pay the bills.

Goddess: Has she ever missed a bill payment?

[Carol starts laughing and says, "Shit…".]

Goddess: Fear gets in the way. Do several things. Increase meditation, hone your ear to my whispers, return to your yoga practice, and stand in *gratitude* for what you have.

Driver: This is so SIMPLE, yet I almost died for this answer. I'm sorry. You've been waiting for me to get out of my own way.

At this point in the session, Goddess has a few more words for Carol and Driver. Before speaking to Sadness, Goddess asked me to have Carol speak to her father's soul, and the session quickly evolved into grief therapy. First, I guided Carol to her peaceful place, and from there asked her to go to a sacred place. Then I incorporated the same profoundly beneficial form of Gestalt role-play described earlier in this chapter, which has helped a number of clients over the years. I suggested that Carol see her father approaching her. She started sobbing immediately, and told him through tears that she missed him. She complained that he left her with an abusive mother. We resume the session here.

> **Father:** I'm so sorry; I didn't know [that your mother was abusive]. I've always been in your heart. Forgive me. I love you. I was there when you buried me.
>
> **Carol:** I miss you. Why did you leave me with a woman who didn't love me?
>
> **Father:** I didn't know.

After some additional dialogue, Carol forgave her father and let him enter the Light. Carol is now free to always remember the good that was in her father, and to be encouraged by his love. When the grief therapy was complete, I returned to parts therapy and asked Goddess to speak.

> **Goddess:** It is now time for Sadness to change her name to Happy Child, and to take a new job. She must now teach Carol how to play.
>
> **Therapist:** Happy Child, do you accept your new name and job from Goddess?
>
> **Happy Child:** I accept!
>
> **Therapist:** Goddess, what other advice do you have?
>
> **Goddess:** Driver gets to merge with Guidance and change her name to Leader. With the power of the Driver partnering with the knowledge of Guidance, Leader will be a powerful part.
>
> **Therapist:** Leader, how do you respond to Goddess?
>
> **Leader:** I accept! Carol will be happier.

After some words of encouragement to each part, all were integrated except for Goddess. The integrated Carol then asked Goddess to talk directly to her.

> **Carol:** Goddess has to talk to me. I want the heartfelt ability to lead and to guide. Where do I take it?
>
> **Therapist:** Goddess, please respond to Carol.
>
> **Goddess:** Listen to your heart and intuition, and you will be listening to me. Stand in my Light. Tell your story and teach. This is so healing on so many levels. This is the soul's healing, not the physical. As the soul is healed, the *life* is healed, and then the body is healed. All the healing shines out to others. This is my command.

On a personal note, Goddess spoke with a tone of voice that projected wisdom and confidence blended with both authority and a deep sense of caring, almost like speaking with an angel. Again, it matters not what you or I think about Goddess. Experts could debate for years over whether that Higher Power part was a figment of Carol's imagination, or a real ego state that was in direct contact with the divine.

In either event, Carol told me that her breakthrough was an answer to prayer, and one that needed to be shared with others. Results speak louder than debates. Perhaps if she shares her own story in written form, she will reveal her real name. The choice is hers. Meanwhile, I deeply appreciate her allowing me to share this profound session in this book with those who seek to understand the potential of the inner mind.

Some weeks later, Carol told me that she has enjoyed some wonderful blessings since this session. She also added, "Thank you so very much, Roy. My wish for you is that this publication will be the foundation for the teaching of parts therapy throughout the world."

My wish for Carol is that her healing of the soul be permanent, helping her to attain her ideal empowerment of mind, body and spirit.

13.5 Exploring spiritual potential—and more

Over the years I've enjoyed the privilege of helping clients access their highest and best wisdom in order to gain further insight regarding their present life path. Common themes include:

- learning to love;
- respecting the freedom of others;
- empowering others;
- appreciating life;
- learning to learn; and
- being tolerant of others.

Often clients are given specific information to help them follow their current life path. Because I am very careful to avoid inappropriate leading, these words come from each client's Higher Power. Sometimes the information is revealed to the conscious mind without being verbalized, leaving me totally unaware of the answers. Finger responses indicate when the client receives an answer to a question.

I believe that spiritual hypnosis must be done with an open mind, and without projecting preconceived opinions into the client. Additionally, such work must be done within the framework of the client's spiritual or philosophical beliefs. Some of the most profound personal breakthroughs I've witnessed through the years have resulted from spiritual hypnosis sessions.

As appropriate, I will continue to use spiritual parts therapy to help people explore their spiritual potential, and perhaps venture farther into the undiscovered country. Much work and research can be done in this area, and I would like to participate in it. When funding makes it possible, I would like to devote a couple of years to facilitating spiritual sessions for various clients who pay for their sessions by giving written permission to publish the results in a book devoted to this topic. It is too important to leave unexplored.

Meanwhile, may those of you who read this book master the art of client-centered parts therapy in order to empower others. When you do so, the client actually becomes his or her own healer, and you are simply the facilitator. Always remember that the client is the one with the power. Your job is to master the art of hypnosis and use your skills to help clients find the keys that unlock their inner power.

This remains true whether the goal is to resolve an inner conflict, or to gain spiritual enlightenment. In either event, we should endeavor to help the client become more empowered. This should be the goal of every hypnotherapist around the world.

When the client comes up with his or her own resolution to a problem during parts therapy or any of its variations, you have facilitated client-centered parts therapy. May this book help you do your part. The rest is up to the client.

You may contact the author by emailing:
alliance@self-empowerment.tv or visit: www.royhunter.com

Bibliography

Baldwin, William J., 1995, *Spirit Releasement Therapy: A Technique Manual*, Headline Books, Inc., Terra Alta, WV. Note: author suggests extreme caution regarding opinions expressed in this book.

Banyan, Calvin D., and Kein, Gerald F., 2001, *Hypnosis and Hypnotherapy: Basic to Advanced Techniques for the Professional*, Abbot Publishing House, Inc., St. Paul, MN.

Beahrs, John O., 1981, *Unity and Multiplicity: Multilevel Consciousness of Self in Hypnosis, Psychiatric Disorder and Mental Health*, Brunner-Routledge, New York, NY.

Boyne, Gil, 1989, *Transforming Therapy: a New Approach to Hypnotherapy*, Westwood Publishing, Glendale, CA.

Bradshaw, John E., 1988, *Bradshaw on the Family: A Revolutionary Way of Self Discovery*, Health Communications, Inc., Deerfield Beach, Florida. Out of print.

Churchill, Randal, 2002, *Regression Hypnotherapy: Transcripts of Transformation*, Transforming Press, Santa Rosa, CA.

Dyak, Miriam, 1999, *The Voice Dialogue Facilitator's Handbook*, L.I.F.E. Energy Press, Seattle, WA.

Emmerson, Gordon, 2003, *Ego State Therapy*, Crown House Publishing, Carmarthen, Wales.

Frederick, Claire, and McNeal, Shirley, 1998, *Inner Strengths: Contemporary Psychotherapy and Hypnosis for Ego-Strengthening*, Lawrence Erlbaum Associates Inc., Mahwah, NJ.

Hogan, Kevin, 2001, *The New Hypnotherapy Handbook*, Network 3000, Eagan, Minnesota.

Hunter, Roy, 2000, *The Art of Hypnotherapy*, 2nd edn, Kendall/Hunt Publishing, Dubuque, Iowa.

Napier, Nancy J., 1990, *Recreating Your SELF: Help for Adult Children of Dysfunctional Families*, W. W. Norton & Company, New York, NY.

Rowan, John, 1993, *Discover Your Subpersonalities*, Routledge, Abingdon, Oxford.

Scheflin, Alan, and Shapiro, Jerrold Lee, 1989, *Trance on Trial*, Guilford Clinical & Experimental Hypnosis Series, Guilford Publications, New York, NY.

Stone, Hal, and Stone, Sidra, 1989, *Embracing Our Selves*, New World Library, Novato, CA.

Tebbetts, Charles, 1997, *Miracles on Demand*, Westwood Publishing Company, Glendale, CA.

Tebbetts, Charles, 1987, *Self-Hypnosis and Other Mind Expanding Techniques*, Westwood Publishing Company, Glendale, CA.

Watkins, John, and Watkins, Helen H., 1997, *Ego States: Theory and Therapy*, W. W. Norton & Company, New York, NY.

Watkins, J. G., and Watkins, H. H., 1979, The theory and practice of ego state therapy. In H. Grayson (Ed.), *Short term approaches to psychotherapy*, Human Sciences Press, New York, NY, pp. 176-220.

Zanuso, Billa, 1986, *The Young Freud: The Origins of Psychoanalysis in Late Nineteenth Century Viennese Culture*, Blackwell Publishers, London. Out of print.

Index

abreactions   31, 73
advance explanation   38, 41,
    147–8
    see also explanation to client
alleged entities   156–63
American Council of Hypnotist
    Examiners   15
asking parts to come to terms of
    agreement, *see under* terms
    of agreement
authority imprint   34

Boyne, Gil   14, 15, 32
Bradshaw, John   8

calling out the part   48, 55–60
calling out other parts   49,
    85–9
casting out parts   156, 159
    see also exorcism
cause, discovering   4, 15–16,
    25, 26–7, 28, 30, 45, 52, 65,
    95
Churchill, Randal   32
concluding the session   117–18
confabulation   26, 98, 159, 161,
    162, 165
conference room   9–10, 51, 63
confirm and summarize terms
    of agreement   49, 106–10
conflicting part   2, 4, 20, 52–3,
    54, 55, 56, 59, 61–2, 65–6,
    69–83 *passim*, 85, 87, 94–5,
    101, 120, 128, 134–5, 143,
    144, 145, 160, 171–2

calling out   58, 88, 94, 142,
    171
    names provided by   65, 74,
    120, 128, 134, 136, 139, 172
    new job for   103
    responses from   68–9
    script for calling out   58
cornerstones of effective
    hypnotherapy   24, 25–9
criticism   54, 81, 90, 94, 143–4,
    152

detours   39, 61–3, 75–6, 93–9,
    101, 104, 108–10
developmental stages   3, 8
discordant parts   89
discovering the purpose   31,
    48, 65–84, 108, 125
discovering the cause   27, 30,
    45, 52
disowned parts   81, 98, 99, 156,
    158
disowned selves   7
dissociative identity disorder
    (DID), *see* multiple
    personalities and multiple
    personality disorder (MPD)
double bind   56, 60
Dyak, Miriam   7

ego parts   3, 4, 7, 8, 152
ego states   3, 6–7, 105, 111,
    150–1
    Freud's   3, 17
ego-state therapy   6–7

eleven-step process   21, 125
  1. Identify the part   48,
    52–3
  2. Gain rapport   48, 53–5
  3. Call out the part   48, 55–60
  4. Thank it for emerging   48,
    60
  5. Discover its purpose   48,
    65–84
  6. Call out other parts   49,
    85–9
  7. Mediate and negotiate   49,
    89–99
  8. Ask parts to come to terms
    of agreement   49, 101–6
  9. Confirm and summarize
    terms of agreement   49,
    106–10
  10. Give suggestions as
    appropriate   49, 111–13
  11. Integrate the parts   49,
    113–16
Emmerson, Gordon   6–7, 33,
    105, 149, 150–1, 156, 167
empowerment   5, 6, 16, 23, 49,
    90, 101, 118, 151, 157, 168,
    180, 181
  self-   28, 174, 176
entities   10, 98–9, 156–63
exorcism   157, 158, 160, 161
explanation to client   38, 40, 41,
    125, 147–8
  see also advance explanation

false memories   26, 31, 33, 46,
    160
Federn, Paul   ix, 3, 16
finger responses   5, 28, 33–6,
    45–6, 56, 61, 65, 181
  parts that use   82–4
  see also ideomotor

flying, fear of   27–8
forgiveness   27, 32, 146, 162
four cornerstones of
    hypnotherapy, *see*
    hypnotherapy objectives

gaining rapport   48, 53–5
Gestalt   3, 7, 10, 32, 146, 174,
    175–6, 179
giving suggestions as
    appropriate   44, 49,
    111–13, 114, 125
grief therapy   146, 174–6, 178

Higher Power   105, 109, 138,
    157–9, 160, 162, 167, 169,
    170, 173, 176, 178, 180, 181
Higher Self   104–5, 106, 157,
    158, 160, 167–8, 169, 175
Hogan, Kevin   10
Hunter, Roy   ix, x, 16
hypnotherapy objectives   23,
    24–9, 30, 116–17
  1. suggestion and imagery
    25–6
  2. discover the cause   25,
    26–7, 30, 45, 52
  3. release   27–8
  4. subconscious relearning
    28–9

identifying the part   48, 52–3,
    125
identifying with someone   34,
    36, 37
ideomotor (responding,
    response, responses)   23,
    26, 33–38
imagery   8, 10, 21, 25–6, 29–30,
    38, 47, 52, 62, 63, 66, 111,
    118, 125, 143, 160

guided   43, 44, 51–2, 112, 116, 118, 126
  open-screen   43, 44
  programmed   43, 44, 51–2
  risk of   51–2
imprint   34, 36
inappropriate leading   26, 27, 32–3, 67, 76–8, 82, 98, 156, 161
inner child   1, 4, 8, 40–1, 56, 66, 69, 81, 134
inner conflict   xi, 1, 2, 5, 6–7, 37, 41, 52, 69, 76, 78, 119, 134
  resolution of   2, 7, 42, 43, 48, 53, 150, 151
inner strength   105, 167
inner wisdom   97, 105–6, 167
integrating the parts   16, 21, 88, 104, 111, 113–16, 124, 133, 153–4

leading and guiding   23, 26, 31
leading questions   46, 68, 86, 95, 98, 160, 161

malevolent state   156
mediation   2, 19–20, 52, 53, 54, 60, 85–99, 112, 159
  negotiation and   4, 49, 89–93
  see also eleven-step process
mistrust   94–6
motivating part   2, 52–3, 54, 55, 59, 61, 63, 73, 77, 80, 83, 85–8, 94–5, 135, 141–2, 143, 145–6, 159, 171, 172
  calling out   52, 53, 55, 58, 59, 62, 65, 75, 85–7, 94, 137, 150, 171

names provided by   66, 67, 86, 121, 129, 137–8, 140, 143, 145, 171
  typical responses from   69, 73
multiple personalities and multiple personality disorder (MPD)   3, 17, 40, 148, 154–6

Napier, Nancy J.   9
National Guild of Hypnotists   15, 16
negative part   98–9, 144, 156, 159, 160
negotiation and mediation, *see under* mediation

offending part   17, 20
  see also conflicting part
outline of parts therapy session   125–6

past event   136
past painful experience   160, 174
personality parts   1, 3, 9, 16, 17, 40, 88
pitfalls   147–65
positive suggestions and affirmations   2, 4, 8, 26, 34, 38, 53, 117
prestige suggestion   24
programmed imagery 43, 44, 51–2
proper preparation   39–50
  establishing finger responses   45
  explanation to client   39–42
  deepening appropriately   42–3

safe place   43–5
verifying hypnotic depth
   45–8
psychodynamics   33–8, 136

Quigley, David   10

rapport   32, 48, 53–5, 57, 60, 67,
   79, 81, 90, 112, 118, 125, 152,
   160, 164
   see also eleven-step process
real or imagined entities, *see*
   alleged entities
regression   26, 27, 30–3, 43, 73,
   136, 153
   hypnotic   8, 23, 26, 27, 30, 31,
      32, 98, 153, 154, 160, 175
   spontaneous   43, 72, 73, 74,
      95, 144, 153
   therapy   15, 23, 30–2, 37, 43,
      73, 77, 156
release   27–8, 32
role-play   3, 10, 32, 92, 107, 113,
   122, 123, 124, 146, 163, 174,
   175–6, 179
   see also Gestalt
Rowan, John   9, 168

safe place   43–5
secondary gain   34, 37, 69, 136
self-punishment   34, 37, 72
selves   3, 7, 8, 9, 168
skipping steps   163
Stone, Hal   7, 8, 156, 168
Stone, Sidra   7, 8, 156, 168
subconscious relearning   3, 25,
   26, 28–9, 30, 116–17, 124
subconscious resistance   3, 26,
   42
subpersonalities   3, 7, 9, 10,
   148, 168

suggestion and imagery   25,
   26, 29, 30, 116, 119, 160
suggestions:
   direct   28, 49, 111–13, 114,
      125, 149
   imagery   25, 26, 29, 30, 116,
      119, 160
   indirect   28, 56, 112, 116
   positive   2, 4, 8, 26, 34, 38, 53,
      117
   prestige suggestion   24

Tebbetts, Charles   ix–x, 2–3, 7,
   10–11, 13–21, 34, 40, 49, 55,
   66, 80, 103, 110, 113, 114,
   127, 149, 150, 152, 164
Tebbetts, Joyce   14–15
terms of agreement   47, 49, 63,
   66, 70, 90, 91, 93, 94, 95, 97,
   98, 101–110, 111, 112, 113,
   114, 118, 123, 142, 148, 150,
   159, 160, 163
   asking parts to come to   49,
      101–6, 125
   confirming and summarizing
      106–10, 125
   thanking part for emerging   65,
      98
therapeutic objectives, *see*
   hypnotherapy objectives
training   7, 15, 23, 24, 29, 153,
   164, 165
   in regression therapy
      30–3

uncooperative part   90, 98–9,
   156, 159
undiscovered country (of inner
   mind)   165, 167–82
unresolved issue   34, 36, 37, 69,
   124

as past grief   174–7 (*see also* grief therapy)
updates   19–21, 56

variations of parts therapy:
  conference room   9–10, 51, 63
  ego-state therapy   6–7
  inner-child work   1, 4, 8, 40–1, 56, 66, 69, 81, 134
  subpersonalities   3, 7, 9, 10, 148, 168

voice dialogue   7–8, 42, 43, 153, 168
voice dialogue, *see under* variations of parts therapy

"W" questions:
  how …?   70–1
  what …?   68–70
  when …?   73
  where …?   74
  who …?   74
  why …?   71–3

USA & Canada orders to:
Crown House Publishing
P.O. Box 2223, Williston, VT 05495-2223, USA
Tel: 877-925-1213, Fax: 802-864-7626
E-mail: info@CHPUS.com
www.CHPUS.com

UK & Rest of World orders to:
The Anglo American Book Company Ltd.
Crown Buildings, Bancyfelin, Carmarthen, Wales SA33 5ND
Tel: +44 (0)1267 211880/211886, Fax: +44 (0)1267 211882
E-mail: books@anglo-american.co.uk
www.anglo-american.co.uk

Australasia orders to:
Footprint Books Pty Ltd.
Unit 4/92A Mona Vale Road, Mona Vale NSW 2103, Australia
Tel: +61 (0) 2 9997 3973, Fax: +61 (0) 2 9997 3185
E-mail: info@footprint.com.au
www.footprint.com.au

Singapore orders to:
Publishers Marketing Services Pte Ltd.
10-C Jalan Ampas #07-01
Ho Seng Lee Flatted Warehouse, Singapore 329513
Tel: +65 6256 5166, Fax: +65 6253 0008
E-mail: info@pms.com.sg
www.pms.com.sg

Malaysia orders to:
Publishers Marketing Services Pte Ltd
Unit 509, Block E, Phileo Damansara 1, Jalan 16/11
46350 Petaling Jaya, Selangor, Malaysia
Tel : 03 7955 3588, Fax : 03 7955 3017
E-mail: pmsmal@po.jaring.my
www.pms.com.sg

South Africa orders to:
Everybody's Books
PO Box 201321, Durban North, 4016, RSA
Tel: +27 (0) 31 569 2229, Fax: +27 (0) 31 569 2234
E-mail: warren@ebbooks.co.za